Empowered Work Teams

IN LONG-TERM CARE

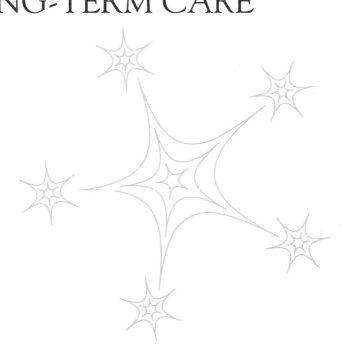

Empowered Work Teams

Strategies for Improving Outcomes for Residents & Staff

IN LONG-TERM CARE

By
Dale E. Yeatts, Ph.D.
Cynthia M. Cready, Ph.D.
Linda S. Noelker, Ph.D.

with invited contributions

Foreword by
Mary Jane Koren, M.D., M.P.H.

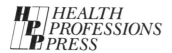
HEALTH PROFESSIONS PRESS

Baltimore • London • Sydney

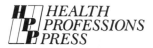
HEALTH PROFESSIONS PRESS

Health Professions Press, Inc.
Post Office Box 10624
Baltimore, Maryland 21285-0624
www.healthpropress.com

Typeset by IPS, Grand Rapids, Michigan.
Manufactured in the United States of America by Maple-Vail Book Manufacturing
Group, York, Pennsylvania.
Cover and interior designs by Mindy Dunn.

Library of Congress Cataloging-in-Publication Data

Yeatts, Dale E., 1952–
Empowered work teams in long-term care : strategies for improving outcomes for residents and staff /
Dale E. Yeatts, Cynthia M. Cready, Linda S. Noelker.
      p. ; cm.
Includes bibliographical references and index.
ISBN 978-1-932529-41-8 (pbk.)
1. Long-term care facilities.   2. Older people—Long-term care.   3. Health care teams.
I. Cready, Cynthia M.   II. Noelker, Linda S.   III. Title.
[DNLM: 1. Long-Term Care—methods.   2. Aged.   3. Patient Care Team—organization & administration.
4. Residential Facilities—organization & administration. WT 31 Y413e 2008]
RA997.Y43 2008
362.16—dc22
2008037375

British Library of Cataloguing-in-Publication data are available from the British Library.

Contents

About the Authors

Dale Yeatts, Ph.D., is Professor of Sociology at the University of North Texas (Denton, TX). His primary areas of study are empowered work teams, gerontology, the workplace, and nursing homes. Dr. Yeatts has received large grants from the National Science Foundation, Commonwealth Fund, and Texas Advanced Research Program to examine "what works" in the case of self-managed work teams in both manufacturing and long-term care settings. His published work has appeared in several books, including *High Performing Self-Managed Work Teams: A Comparison of Theory to Practice*, and in academic and professional journals, including *The Gerontologist* and *Journal of Gerontological Nursing*.

Cynthia M. Cready, Ph.D., is Associate Professor of Sociology at the University of North Texas (Denton, TX). Her research interests include long-term care of elders, family, and racial/ethnic differentiation and inequality. Her articles on these topics have been published in a variety of journals, including *The Gerontologist*, *The Milbank Quarterly*, *Health Services Research*, *Journal of Marriage and the Family*, *Social Science Quarterly*, and others.

Linda S. Noelker, Ph.D., is the Senior Vice President for Planning and Organizational Resources and the Director of the Katz Policy Institute at the Benjamin Rose Institute (Cleveland, OH). Dr. Noelker received her graduate degrees from Case Western Reserve University where she is an Adjunct Professor of Sociology. She is the former Editor-in-Chief of *The Gerontologist*, the leading scientific journal in applied aging research, practice, and policy. Dr. Noelker holds leadership positions in the American Society on Aging and the Gerontological Society of America, the two major professional societies in the field of aging. She received the 2005 American Society on Aging Award for exemplary contributions to the field of gerontology and the 2005 Distinguished Career in Gerontology Award from the Behavioral and Social Sciences section of the Gerontological Society of America. Throughout her career, she has conducted research on the nature and effects of family care for frail elders, patterns of service use by older adults and their family caregivers, and sources of stress and job satisfaction among direct care workers.

Contributors

Keith A. Anderson, Ph.D.
Assistant Professor
The Ohio State University
College of Social Work
1947 N. College Road
Columbus, OH 43215-1162

Farida K. Ejaz, Ph.D.
Benjamin Rose Institute
11900 Fairhill Road, Suite 300
Cleveland, OH 44120-1053

Joseph E. Gaugler, Ph.D.
Associate Professor
School of Nursing, Center on Aging
Coordinator for Research Initiatives
Center for Gerontological Nursing
University of Minnesota
6-153 Weaver-Densford Hall 1331
308 Harvard Street S.E.
Minneapolis, MN 55455

Mauro Hernandez, Ph.D., CEO
Concepts in Community Living, Inc.
15900 S.E. 82nd Drive
Clackamas, OR 97015

Mary Jane Koren, M.D., M.P.H.
Assistant Vice President
The Commonwealth Fund
One East 75th Street
New York, NY 10021

Heather L. Menne, Ph.D.
Benjamin Rose Institute
11900 Fairhill Road, Suite 300
Cleveland, OH 44120-1053

Katherina A. Nikzad
Hartford Doctoral Fellow
Graduate Center for Gerontology
University of Kentucky
306 Wethington Health Sciences
    Building
900 South Limestone
Lexington, KY 40536-0200

Jude Rabig, RN, Ph.D.
Rabig Consulting
251 East 77th Street 2B
New York, NY 10021

Acknowledgments

Much of the research and experience reported in this book was funded by the Commonwealth Fund, a private independent foundation based in New York City. We wish to thank all those at the Commonwealth Fund who supported us in our research efforts, including Stephen Schoenbaum, Mary Jane Koren, Ann Marie Audet, and Clare Churchouse. Of course, the views presented are our own and not necessarily those of the Commonwealth Fund or its directors, officers, or staff.

We also want to thank the executives, managers, nurses, and direct care workers of C.C. Young, Christian Care Centers, Evangelical Lutheran Good Samaritan Society, Mariner Health Care, Nexion Health, and Pacific Retirement Services, who were willing to try something new by implementing empowered work teams.

Finally, we would like to thank those who served in an advisory group that provided direction at the beginning of the empowerment project, including Drs. Barbara Bowers, Susan Cohen, Susan Eaton, and Robyn Stone.

Foreword

The baby boom generation has been the pig in the python throughout its existence—first for schools, then housing, and, as this generation approaches retirement age, for long-term care (LTC) services. But even before the baby boomers hit 85, the age at which support for diminishing function becomes ever more important, the reality of smaller families, more working women, and families that are geographically separated is ratcheting up the urgency that we face to ensure an array of adequate, high-quality LTC services that meet the needs of today's older adults.

Circumstances permitting, receiving care in one's own home is preferred to care in a residential facility. Hence the emphasis on the part of policy makers to afford better access to home- and community-based services. Nevertheless, the combination of extreme frailty, worsening chronic conditions, and lack of sufficient informal supports means that for many older adults nursing homes (NHs) will continue to be an important component of the LTC system. NHs, however, must address numerous issues concerning the quality of care they provide. A survey by the Kaiser Family Foundation found that the vast majority of those surveyed were concerned about NH quality. Also, the Centers for Medicare and Medicaid Services identified roughly one quarter of all NHs in the United States as having excessive rates of pressure ulcers and restraints.

Because LTC is a high-touch, not high-tech field, quality of care is inextricably linked to the number and skill level of staff, particularly the hands-on staff, or *direct care workers* (DCW). This is especially the case in NHs, where it is the DCW (also referred to as a certified nursing assistant or CNA) who attends to the physical needs of residents and, as a result, contributes greatly to the quality of life of residents. The relationship a NH resident has with his or her nursing assistant is one of the most important contributors to overall comfort and satisfaction.

Unfortunately, workforce is one of the major problems facing the LTC field—we cannot have a high-performing LTC system without employees. While employee shortages exist at all levels, from administrators to CNAs, the need for more DCWs is one of the most pressing concerns providers face. Oddly enough, it is this very level of employee, the direct care worker, that is the most undervalued. CNAs are too often viewed as expendable and interchangeable. They are paid a lowly wage at the cost of a high turnover rate, which, depending on the source of the data, is often reported as 70% annually or higher in NHs. This cost is simply factored into the price of doing business. Recruiting and retaining workers in such an environment is difficult in the extreme. When asked, however, CNAs will often say they love the work but hate the job. Too often regarded as escapees from the fast-food industry, they are far more often dedicated workers with a commitment to caring for the most vulnerable and compromised among older adults. The NH industry has only itself to blame for the situation.

There are a number of factors, easily within the control of providers, that make working as a DCW or CNA such an unappealing job, and only one of those is compensation. Health care organizations tend to be hierarchical, a characteristic that extends to its associated professions, including nursing. Within NHs there is no doubt as to who is at the bottom of the pecking order—CNAs rank dead last. Their expertise is disregarded by their professional nursing colleagues and their creativity untapped by management. Rarely are they valued as a vital resource within their facility. Instead they are seen as a cost center and as a pool of unskilled workers to be managed and supervised by those above them.

This book is an antidote to the prevailing and toxic situation that exists in all too many NHs today. It provides a thoughtful examination of the problem, including its historical antecedents, as well as a better understanding of the sociologic factors at play in today's LTC settings. It is also a practical and much-needed guide for developing a new course. If our aging parents (and eventually we ourselves) are to be well cared for, we cannot continue to do business as usual.

The concept of teams has been shown to be effective in other industries and it is particularly apt in the LTC setting, where a team effort has to exist if the work of caring for older adults is to be done well. To date, however, teams in LTC have more often been used to bring different disciplines together to collectively work on complex care challenges or as a way of connecting different levels within a professional hierarchy. This book focuses instead on peer teams. It shows NHs how to help DCWs create self-managed teams that harvest and share the skills and knowledge present in the group. Such teams give otherwise disenfranchised individual workers a collective voice to make their needs for better training or particular resources known to management. Also, as DCWs are recognized as expert in what they do and are given some control over their work, they gain status within the organization and pride in their accomplishments. The challenge of maintaining a sufficient staff of well-trained workers will not be magically solved by the creation of empowered work teams. When DCWs, however, are finally given the job they want in order to do the work they love, more than half the battle will have been won.

Mary Jane Koren, M.D., M.P.H.
Assistant Vice President
The Commonwealth Fund, New York

Preface

The use of empowered work teams (EWTs) in long-term care settings stems from earlier lessons learned by managers of manufacturing corporations. In the last quarter of the 20th century, corporations began experiencing intense international competition. As managers looked for ways to compete, one solution they found was better use of their human resources. This included organizing their nonmanagement employees into teams and then allowing the teams to make decisions regarding how to improve work processes as well as other aspects of their work.

Managers first began experimenting with the team approach by having team members meet once a week with management to share their thoughts on how to improve the work process. These came to be known as *quality circles*. The workers shared ways to reduce steps in the work process, improve efficiency in the steps, and allow the workers to be more efficient when performing the steps, all of which typically resulted in financial savings. Further, employees appreciated being asked for their opinions so that job attitudes improved as well.

As quality circles became more entrenched in the workplace, managers began allowing the nonmanagement teams to become more involved in the decision-making process where the decisions to be made involved their work. In this way, workplace decisions were made by or highly influenced by those who were actually doing the work, those with firsthand knowledge. These teams came to be known as *self-directed* or *self-managed* work teams and later as *empowered* work teams.

It was at this time that the lead author, Dale Yeatts, began to gain knowledge and experience with EWTs. As a budding sociologist, he had two major areas of study: industrial sociology and social gerontology, with multiple publications in both areas. Clearly, the study of EWTs fit within the field of industrial sociology. Yeatts initially obtained a grant to evaluate how effective EWTs are in the workplace. This was followed by a second grant to identify those factors most important to the success of the EWTs. This included identifying what works and what doesn't work when using empowered teams in large organizations, such as Texas Instruments or Boeing.

As the study and knowledge of EWTs evolved, Yeatts began to see a potential link between EWTs and his study of gerontology and, in particular, long-term care. It was clear that nursing homes in general were experiencing difficulties providing high quality care. Like the manufacturing sector, nursing homes were being asked to provide higher quality service with fewer resources. At the same time, they were experiencing high staff turnover. Yeatts concluded that perhaps the use of EWTs in nursing homes, in the form of direct care worker (DCW) teams, would allow for better communication among the DCWs and between the DCWs and nurses, would allow for more firsthand knowledge to be applied to decisions about the work process and residents, and might improve job attitudes and consequently reduce staff turnover.

Yeatts along with the book's second author, Cynthia Cready, received a grant to establish EWTs in five nursing homes, with five additional nursing homes used as a comparison group. The results of their work, along with that of the third author, Linda Noelker, and others are discussed in this book. The authors identify the advantages that have been gained from using EWTs in nursing homes, the potential advantages for home care and assisted living settings, and the steps that can be followed in order to create these teams so that the EWTs reach their full potential.

Almost all recent initiatives in long-term care have encouraged more empowerment of DCWs. Unfortunately, most of these initiatives provide no clear directions on how to make this happen. This book helps to fill that gap in the knowledge base. As the empowerment of DCWs grows in long-term care and becomes more routine, the day-to-day care of residents will improve as will the attitudes of the direct care workers.

We dedicate this book to Dr. Hiram Friedsam,
who passed on in 2007 after a long life of service
to older Americans and the field of gerontology.

PART I

Why Create Empowered Work Teams in Long-Term Care?

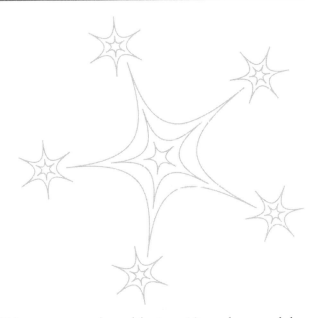

Empowered work teams (EWTs) are groups of roughly 4 to 10 employees of the same rank or level (e.g., all computer board assemblers or all direct care workers). This is different from interdisciplinary work teams, made up of people with differing job titles and levels (e.g., social worker, nurse, and physician). Those in an EWT are responsible for directing some or most aspects of their work, including planning and scheduling who will do what, ordering supplies as needed, and monitoring the team's performance. At the same time, the employees are still responsible for performing the technical aspects of their work, whether it is assembling computer boards to be installed in smart bombs or helping residents to the dining hall (Johnson & Johnson, 1994; Wellins, Byham, & Dixon, 1994; Yeatts & Hyten, 1998).

The use of EWTs first occurred in manufacturing settings and has spread widely. Numerous studies have shown that such teams improve an employee's performance and attitude and reduce turnover and absenteeism. However, the research also indicates that these effects are contingent on successful implementation of the teams. And the research has taken place primarily in manufacturing settings.

More recently, EWTs have been introduced into service and health care settings. Long-term care (LTC) appears to be particularly well suited for EWTs. Traditionally LTC has used a medical model, which is characterized by a rigid hierarchical structure that leaves little room for those providing direct service to contribute to management decisions. It has been suggested that the resulting institutional culture may contribute to poor employee performance, low satisfaction among direct care workers, and exceptionally high turnover, often between 60% and 80% a year, in nursing homes (NHs) (Binstock & Spector, 1997; Cohen-Mansfield, 1997; Halbur, 1986; Packer-Tursman, 1996). Research in the manufacturing industry and some in health care suggests that allowing those who actually do the hands-on work (e.g., direct care workers) to participate in decision making will result in better decisions being made, more satisfied employees, and lower turnover and absenteeism.

Updating management strategies has been recognized for some time as a way to improve resident care. In the 1980s Congress commissioned a study by the Institute of Medicine to determine how best to improve the quality of NH care. This study concluded that the resident care provided was a direct result of how LTC employees are managed (Heiselman & Noelker, 1991; Institute of Medicine, 1986). In the 1990s, Binstock and Spector (1997) conducted an in-depth study funded by the Agency for Health Care Policy and Research to identify the five highest-priority areas for research to improve LTC. One of the five areas they identified was management practices. They found that there was a lack of knowledge among NH administrators regarding effective strategies for managing NH staff and that this appeared to be having detrimental effects on the direct care provided to residents (see also Davis, 1991). More recently, the U.S. Centers for Medicare and Medicaid Services have recognized the need to move beyond the medical model for managing LTC facilities. To assist LTC providers, they have set an expectation that quality improvement organizations across the country will help LTC providers transition from a medical model of care to a more person-centered model.

The result has been the introduction of a variety of initiatives. For example, the Pioneer Network was organized in the 1990s with the purpose of identifying "deep systematic change" that will allow a "person-centered" focus of care (Fagan, 2003, p. 125). Members of this network include practitioners, researchers, educators, and other professionals who seek to find alternatives to the strictly medical model. In 1992 the Eden Alternative was developed by Thomas and Thomas (Thomas, 1994, 2006) to encourage a more homelike environment in the NH, and a decade later Thomas and his colleagues introduced the promising concept of Green Houses that provide a structural alternative in the form of specially designed houses for older adults (Keane, 2004). In 1994, another approach, the Wellspring Model, was established to encourage NHs to work together to teach line staff best clinical practices and to change the typical NH culture of control (Kehoe & Heesch, 2003; Reinhard & Stone, 2001). In 2001, the Learn, Empower, Achieve, and Produce (LEAP) initiative was under way to change how the NH workforce was viewed and treated by NH management (Hollinger-Smith, 2003; Hollinger-Smith, Ortigara, & Lindeman, 2001). In a more recent development, Grant and Norton (2003) identified various stages that NHs are expected to go through in the process of culture change. Additional recent initiatives include those by Gilster, Accorinti, and Dalessandro (2002, Pillemer, Suitor, and Wethington et al. (2003), Rosen et al. (2005), and Shields (2004).

One characteristic typically found as a component of these and other person-centered initiatives has been the empowering of direct care staff (also called front-line staff). It is reasoned that direct care workers have the most knowledge about residents; they know better than any other employees the likes and dislikes of residents. This might include what they want when they wake up in the morning (e.g., a glass of water or the newspaper), where they prefer to go during the day, and what they want to wear when they go to bed at night. Consequently, the direct care workers are in the best position to make decisions that are directly related to day-to-day resident care (Beck, Ortigara, Mercer, & Shue, 1999).

A second major reason for introducing EWTs into LTC has been offered by Cohen-Mansfield and Noelker (2000, p. 52). They note that "projections indicate there will be a shortage of nursing assistants that will reach crisis proportions in coming years. This will be the direct result of the increasing elderly population, particularly among the oldest-old (those 85 and over) who make the greatest use of nursing home care." Although the LTC workforce must grow nearly 70% in the first decade of the 21st century, the U.S. labor force is projected to grow at a rate of only 1.2% annually (Cohen-Mansfield, 1997). Unless there is some way of attracting new NH employees, there will not be adequate staff available to provide care. One means of attracting new NH employees is a management strategy that focuses on making the work more attractive, such as by allowing employees to have a voice in management decisions that are related to their work.

While the need for LTC employees is increasing, those who currently work in LTC are quitting at an alarming rate and show high levels of absenteeism (De-Francis, 2002; Eaton, 2000). Turnover rates among NH employees usually range from 40% to 75%, with some reaching 500% (Banaszak-Holl & Hines, 1996; Caudill & Patrick, 1991–1992; Kane, 2001). Such high turnover rates along with high absenteeism negatively affect continuity of care and the establishment of personal relationships between direct care workers and residents. These relationships have been found to be important to high-quality care (Caudill & Patrick, 1991–1992; Waxman, Carner, & Berkenstock, 1984). More specifically, long tenure typically results in the LTC employees becoming more familiar with the residents and their likes and dislikes. This results in higher performance outcomes, particularly when measured in terms of customer (e.g., resident) satisfaction. Similarly, high levels of absenteeism reduce the continuity of care, and as a result residents are served by many different employees, many of whom are unfamiliar with their preferences (Caudill & Patrick, 1991–1992).

Furthermore, turnover has the added problem of cost, because the LTC facility must constantly advertise for new employees and provide orientation training. A study of NH staff turnover by Caudill and Patrick (1991–1992) reveals that NH facilities can pay more than $7,000 per RN replacement and more than $2,000 to replace a certified nurse aide (Cohen-Mansfield, 1997).

One way to retain employees is to make their jobs more desirable (Wiener, 2002). Unfortunately, traditional LTC management strategies do a very poor job of this. Research suggests that appropriately implemented EWTs can make the job

of a direct care worker more desirable. Successful implementation entails attention to staff training, team design, and, most importantly, management support.

Chapter 1 defines empowerment and types of EWTs, provides a brief review
of the large body of research that has been conducted in the manufacturing setting
to determine the effects of empowering nonmanagement staff, and reviews factors
important to EWT success. Chapter 2 provides a picture of how EWTs are currently operating in NHs. Chapters 3 and 4 describe how EWTs might be used in
assisted living facilities and home care settings.

What We Know About Empowered Work Teams in Non–Long-Term Care Settings
Lessons Learned

The term *employee empowerment* has a variety of meanings and implications. From a psychological perspective, empowerment is "a subjective state of mind whereby an employee perceives that he or she is exercising efficacious control over meaningful work" (Potterfield, 1999, p. 51). Thus empowered people find meaning in their work through an enhanced sense of control and participation in decision making, thereby influencing and determining desired outcomes. From a relational perspective, empowerment is the "relocation of power from the upper levels of the organizational hierarchy to the lower levels of rank-and-file workers" (Potterfield, 1999, p. 52). This relational perspective focuses more on the structure of the organization and the power relationships between groups. In this view, empowered people share power and information, and communication flows freely within the hierarchy of the organization, resulting in enhanced service and a greater sense of ownership among workers.

Traditionally, most workplaces and businesses, including long-term care (LTC), have been structured in a pyramid shape, with a small number of high-level decision makers at the top of the pyramid and a large number of workers forming the base of the pyramid. Work is organized by managers and dictated to the workers in a clearly and often narrowly defined fashion. Information in the pyramid structure flows downward, and rarely do workers have input into managerial decisions. This structure allows a high level of managerial control and facilitates the training and replacement of lower-echelon workers. As one might imagine, this structure does not promote the empowerment of workers; rather, it precludes workers from participating in decision making and effecting change in work processes (Potterfield, 1999).

In contrast, the organizational structures of empowered workplaces are shaped like stars, circular networks, spider webs, or inverted pyramids. Decisions are made and work is organized through the free flow of information and input between upper-echelon managers and lower-echelon direct care workers (e.g., nurses, home health aides). Empowered workplaces encourage creativity and innovation in direct care workers to enable both the workers and the overall organization to perform at the highest possible level. Thus all levels of workers share in decision-making processes and ultimately in the success of the organization (Quinn, 1992).

The use of empowered work teams (EWTs) has become a staple for many U.S. corporations that have experienced intense international competition since the last quarter of the 20th century. This competition has created a growing need to find new ways of reducing expenses while maintaining or increasing productivity and quality. A comparable urgency can be seen in the current crisis in LTC, where managers are being asked to provide higher-quality care with fewer resources.

Competition has led many executives to reexamine their organizations' structures and processes, particularly the use of human resources. A growing number of executives have concluded that they could make better use of their nonmanagement employees by allowing them to participate in management decisions related to their work (Black & Gregersen, 1997; Donovan, 1988, 1989; Henricks, 1997; Lawler, 1986, 1992).

The idea of using the knowledge of nonmanagement workers to improve the organization's performance was not new. W. Edwards Deming (1993) presented the idea to a number of U.S. corporate executives in the 1960s, but at that time they were not in a mood to listen, given the lack of competition and hence the lack of desire to make changes. However, Deming found that Japanese corporate executives were more than ready to listen to his approach to management, which included taking advantage of the firsthand knowledge that nonmanagement employees have. As a result, Japanese businesses gained a competitive advantage in several industries.

RATIONALE FOR EMPOWERING EMPLOYEES

The rationale for involving workers in decision making comes from at least three different schools of thought. Cognitive models suggest that it is the sharing of information at all levels of the organization that is the key. Employee participation in decision making improves performance because it enhances the flow and use of important information within the organization (Anthony, 1978; Frost, Wakely, & Ruh, 1974; Kren, 1992; Pasmore & Purser, 1993).

The human relations school argues that participation is effective because it meets higher-order employee needs, such as self-expression, respect, and independence, which in turn increases morale, satisfaction, and commitment and reduces labor turnover and absenteeism (Bouckaert, 1999; Cummings, 1978; Hackman & Oldham, 1976; Hyman & Mason, 1995; Lawler, 1986; Likert, 1967). Employee involvement theory has grown out of this school and emphasizes giving power to nonmanagement employees in the form of information, rewards, and training, with the result being high employee performance and satisfaction (Lawler, 1986).

Finally, contingency models argue that no one theoretical explanation holds across the wide variety of individuals and situations. Instead, the effects of employee participation on performance and satisfaction are contingent on the specific industry, people, and situations involved (Anderson, 1992; Kelly, 1991; Schuster et al., 1997; Singer, 1974; Yeatts & Hyten, 1998).

WHAT IS EMPLOYEE EMPOWERMENT?

Employee empowerment, found in EWTs and other management strategies, has come to mean more than simply the employees' autonomy in making decisions or participation in decision making. However, most research that has been done, particularly in the manufacturing setting, has used these features as the conceptual framework for employee empowerment. More recently, employee empowerment has been defined in somewhat different ways, depending on the researchers involved.

Kirkman and Rosen (1999) and others view employee empowerment as a combination of four factors. In addition to perceiving autonomy on the job, the employee perceives her work to be meaningful and to have important impacts, and the employee feels highly competent in doing the work. These researchers believe a combination of these factors instills a feeling of empowerment (see also Bandura, 1997; Ford & Fottler, 1995; Spreitzer, 1995; Spreitzer, Kizilos, & Nason, 1997; Thomas & Velthouse, 1990).

Kanter (1993) also defines employee empowerment as having four primary components, although hers are somewhat different. These include access to information necessary to do the job, the opportunity to learn and grow, the resources needed for the job, and workplace support. Two of these—access to information and necessary resources—are similar to Kirkman and Rosen's focus on competence, and the opportunity to learn and grow can be viewed as similar to Kirkman and Rosen's emphasis on meaningfulness and impact of the work. Feelings of support and feelings of autonomy also have similarities.

WHAT ARE EWTS?

As international competition increased in the 1970s and 1980s, managers in the United States began searching for ways to improve performance. Many turned to Deming's philosophy, and this often led them to establish quality circles. These are groups of nonmanagement employees who meet weekly with a manager so that the manager can learn potential ways of improving the organization's processes. Research has shown that quality circles can be very effective at first, but their effectiveness appears to drop over time (Griffin, 1988).

The organization of employees into quality circles eventually gave way to the establishment of "autonomous work groups." These were groups made up exclusively of nonmanagement employees who began to think of themselves as a team and were given the opportunity to participate in decision making or in some cases to make decisions about their work. As these groups gained autonomy, they came to be called "self-directed teams." And as these teams gained decision-making authority, some began to call them "self-managed work teams." Unfortunately, the use of these terms by researchers and managers has not been consistent. Consequently, the more general term "empowered work teams" avoids any misunderstandings because it does not imply a specific level of empowerment.

As noted in the introduction to Part I, an EWT typically consists of 4 to 10 employees of the same rank or level who are responsible for managing some or most aspects of their work, including planning and scheduling who will do what, ordering supplies, and monitoring the team's performance. At the same time, the employees are still responsible for performing the technical duties of their jobs (Johnson & Johnson, 1994; Wellins, Byham, & Dixon, 1994; Yeatts & Hyten, 1998).

Most recently, the practice of empowering employees has spread beyond manufacturing settings to other areas such as the social service and health care industries. These unique work settings are establishing their own forms of work teams that allow employee empowerment. For example, in nursing homes EWTs typically are made up of direct care workers, most of whom are certified nursing assistants. Again, these are different from interdisciplinary work teams, made up of people with differing job titles and levels (e.g., social worker, nurse, physician). EWTs in nursing homes typically are authorized to make some decisions related to their work and routinely provide input to nurse management before management decisions are made. However, EWTs in nursing homes tend to be different from those in manufacturing in that the team members have less decision-making authority, in part because of government regulations that prevent social service and health care employees from making particular types of decisions. But this appears also to reflect the hierarchical nature of the health care system, which does not encourage participation of nonmanagement employees.

EFFECTS OF EMPOWERED WORK TEAMS:
A REVIEW OF RESEARCH IN MANUFACTURING

Scientific research on EWTs has occurred almost exclusively in the manufacturing industry. These studies suggest that under the right circumstances manufacturing employees who are allowed to participate in management decisions perform at a higher level, have higher job satisfaction, and have lower turnover and absenteeism than do employees in a more traditional manufacturing environment where employee participation is not sought or allowed (Hitchcock & Willard, 1995; Ray & Bronstein, 1995; Shonk, 1992; Wellins et al., 1994; Yeatts & Hyten, 1998).

Research has also found that the quality of work often improves when direct care workers become involved in management decisions (Hitchcock & Willard, 1995; Wellins et al., 1994; Yeatts & Hyten, 1998). This is because those making the decisions—the team members—are the most knowledgeable about the work and about those performing the work. This has been found to be true even where the formal education of the employees is very low (Lawler, 1986; Macy, Peterson, & Norton, 1989; Pasmore, Francis, Haldeman, & Shani, 1982; Wellins et al., 1994).

Furthermore, it has been shown that the team members in EWTs often are able to consider both social and technical factors more effectively than managers or engineers. In more traditional settings, decisions often are made by engineers or managers who either do not consider social factors (e.g., who works best with whom) or are less familiar with the social factors than are the team members who work side by side. Similarly, engineers and managers sometimes are less familiar with the technical aspects of the work because they often lack the advantage of firsthand knowledge (Anthony, 1978; Hackman, 1978; Lawler, 1986; Myers, 1991; Susman, 1979).

Finally, EWTs have also been found to reduce employee turnover because they increase job satisfaction and because team members become increasingly committed to the decisions their team makes. If an employee is told how to do a particular task but the employee does not believe the procedures are the best available, the employee will carry out the task with some reservation. However, if the employee has been involved in designing the procedure to be used and believes it to be the best available, the employee will perform the task more enthusiastically and routinely.

Although many studies show the positive effects of EWTs, a number of scientific studies have found few, none, or even negative effects. The most common reason given is that the EWTs were not established in a way that allowed them to be successful. For example, team members may not have been given adequate resources (e.g., equipment, tools) to do the work. Or the employees on the team may not have had all the knowledge, skill, and ability needed to do the work (e.g., training in how to schedule). These studies suggest that when certain features are not present to support the EWT, the effects of the EWT can be negligible or even negative (Nurick, 1982; Tjosvold, 1986; Varney, 1989; Yeatts & Hyten, 1998). Therefore, to understand the impacts of EWTs, one must also consider the factors that contribute to a team's performance.

CHARACTERISTICS OF AN EFFECTIVE EMPOWERED WORK TEAM

Many theoretical models have been presented to highlight the most important characteristics affecting an EWT's performance (see Campion, Medsker, & Higgs, 1993; Cohen, 1994; Gladstein, 1984; Hackman, 1988; McGrath, 1964; Pearce & Ravlin, 1987; Salas, Dickinson, Converse, & Tannenbaum, 1992; Sundstrom, De Meuse, & Futrell, 1990; Tannenbaum, Beard, & Salas, 1992; Yeatts & Hyten, 1998). Most of these include an input–process–output framework. In the simplest model, the most important factors include those related to the work process itself, the interpersonal processes, the team design, the environment of the team, and the characteristics of the team members (Figure 1.1). These factors are discussed briefly after a discussion of EWT performance.

Measuring Empowered Work Team Performance

The performance of EWTs in manufacturing has been viewed as the team's ability to satisfy its customers in terms of the quantity and quality of a product and the team's timeliness and overall costs (Gladstein, 1984; McGrath, 1964; Nieva, Fleishman, & Rieck, 1978). Yeatts and Hyten (1998, pp. 51-52) cite a memorandum from a manager addressing the importance of customer satisfaction: "It is critical that each team take responsibility for satisfying their customers. We will be encouraging them to visit their customers, whether that means other teams, engi-

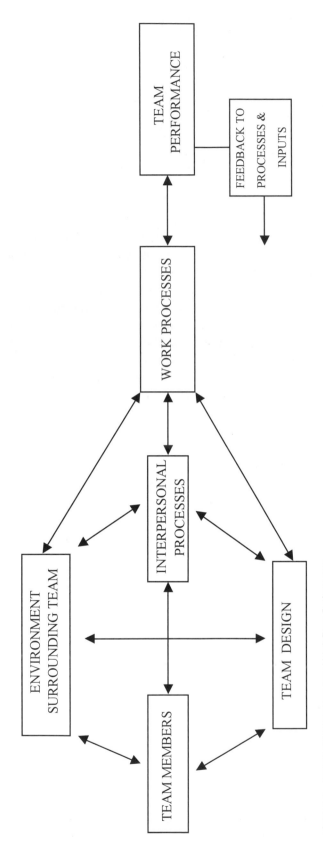

Figure 1.1. Factors Affecting Empowered Work Team Performance.

neers, managers, etc., to learn their customers' 'care-abouts.' Measuring customer satisfaction is a challenge. We will help the teams explore alternatives for measuring and improving this important metric."

Team performance has also been measured as the economic viability of the team (Yeatts & Hyten, 1998), that is, the team's ability to function at a profit for the larger organization. If the team is providing a high-quality product, but it costs more to produce the product than the income generated from it, the team's performance is considered problematic.

Of particular importance for EWTs in LTC is customer service. Unfortunately, outside the laboratory setting it is often difficult to identify exactly what good customer service is (Hackman, 1990). This holds true even when we can measure specific outputs, such as the number of people served, the number of complaints or compliments received, or the amount of time needed to do a task. The questions that must be asked when considering these measures include "Is team performance high when the team produces more than most similar teams?" "If one team serves more residents in less time, does that constitute higher performance?" The answer to these is clearly "no" if the customer is dissatisfied with the service or the cost of providing the service is too high. Are teams that produce a higher-quality service higher-performing teams? Again, the answer is clearly "no" if the customer would prefer to pay less and receive less quality.

Thus quantitative criteria that simply measure levels of productivity or quality are not necessarily good indicators of the team's performance. Simple quantitative measures may not validly indicate how well a team has done its work because such measures do not consider the preferences of the team's customers or the economic viability of the team.

The Work Process

Several researchers conclude that the most important factors directly affecting a team's performance are work process factors (Figure 1.1; Hackman, 1988; Yeatts & Hyten, 1998). These include the level of individual effort applied to the work, the skill and knowledge applied to the work, and the procedures used to do the work. All other factors are less important than what occurs as the work is done. For example, a worker may have a high level of skill and knowledge resulting from a well-designed training program (an environmental characteristic), but if this skill and knowledge are not actually applied to the work, then they are of little value. Similarly, a team may have a well-designed procedure for accomplishing a particular task (a team design factor), but if the team uses a different procedure to accomplish the task, then the well-designed procedure is of little value. And an employee may be highly motivated to do the work (a team member characteristic), but if something is preventing him or her from doing the work effectively (e.g., he or she does not know the best procedure for accomplishing the task), then the high level of motivation is of little value.

Thus the work process is what actually happens as the work is done: the actual amount of effort applied to the work, the actual skills and knowledge used, and the actual procedures used. All other factors are important in that they enhance or inhibit the work process.

Interpersonal Processes

Many theorists conclude that team member interactions are the most important factors affecting work team performance (Ancona & Caldwell, 1992; Brightman, 1988; Holt, 1990; Jewell & Reitz, 1988; Johnson & Johnson, 1994; Katz & Kahn, 1966; Schindler & Thomas, 1993; Tjosvold, 1986). Team member interactions are personal interactions that occur between team members and between team members and people outside the team. Team member interactions that have received the most attention include communication, coordination, cooperation, conflict, cohesion, commitment, and trust. Many theorists view these as intermediate factors between the input and output factors and in so doing typically ignore the effects of the team's work processes. Although interpersonal processes are closely tied to work processes, research suggests that they are not the same (Hackman, 1990; Yeatts & Hyten, 1998).

An examination of the relationship between team member interactions and work processes suggests that interpersonal processes can have a variety of positive and negative effects (Gladstein, 1984; Heiselman & Noelker, 1991; Pearce & Ravlin, 1987; Sundstrom et al., 1990; Tannenbaum et al., 1992). For example, accurate and frequent communication and coordination have been found to result in the team designing and using the most appropriate work procedures (Ancona & Caldwell, 1992; Neuhaus, 1990; Yeatts & Hyten, 1998). Similarly, studies show that high cohesion, cooperation, and commitment can result in higher effort and more knowledge and skill being applied to the work as team members work together and combine their talents. Low cohesion can have negative impacts on effort applied to the work as employees spend large amounts of time struggling to reach agreements (Holt, 1990; Seashore, 1954; Yeatts & Hyten, 1998).

The Team's Environment

Several theorists emphasize the environment as particularly important to an EWT's performance (Ancona & Caldwell, 1992; Becker-Reems, 1994; Pearce & Ravlin, 1987; Sundstrom et al., 1990; Wetherbe, 1991). The environment includes factors within the organization but outside the team and factors outside the organization. Influential factors proposed to exist within the organization include the organization's culture, support from management, feedback, and organizational systems for training, information exchange, performance assessment, and reward distribution. Important environmental factors outside the organization include customer characteristics, government regulations, the state of the economy, societal culture, and the unemployment rate (Pearce & Ravlin, 1987; Sundstrom et al., 1990). These factors outside the organization have received much less attention from researchers, in part because of difficulties in obtaining the data needed for sophisticated statistical analyses.

The environmental factors receiving the most attention from researchers appear to be internal factors related to the organization's reward and information systems, feedback, and management support. For example, it has been found that correct and timely information helps EWT members select the most appropriate procedures for doing the work (Ancona & Caldwell, 1992; Becker-Reems, 1994; Wetherbe, 1991; Yeatts & Hyten, 1998). Reward systems designed for EWTs have been shown to increase team member effort (Gross, 1995; Lawler, 1989; Sims & Manz, 1994).

An environmental characteristic that is particularly unique to LTC is the characteristics of the customers or clients. Customer characteristics receive little attention among those who have studied EWT performance in manufacturing settings. In manufacturing settings the customer often is another organization or perhaps another team within the same organization. Characteristics of such customers rarely are treated as affecting the EWT's performance. However, when the EWT's customers are a group of clients or a group of residents in a nursing home or assisted living facility, customer characteristics may have a profound influence on the EWT's work processes and performance. For example, the residents' health conditions (e.g., disabilities, discomfort) and health practices (e.g., self-care, risky behaviors) can be expected to affect the EWT's work processes and, in particular, the team's procedures for doing the work. Other important resident characteristics might include the availability of informal care and support and demographic characteristics (e.g., age, gender, heredity).

Team Design Factors

Some researchers focus almost exclusively on an EWT's design to explain EWT performance. Team design factors that receive attention include the size of the team, the extent of the team's empowerment, goal clarity, role conflict, the team's decision-making processes, and the team's stability in terms of personnel (Anderson & McDaniel, 1998; Barber & Iwai, 1996; Beyerlein & Johnson, 1994; Hitchcock & Willard, 1995; Lekan-Rutledge, Palmer, & Belyea, 1998; Manz & Sims, 1987; Orsburn, Moran, Musselwhite, Zenger, & Perrin, 1990; Ray & Bronstein, 1995; Rennecker, 1996).

The effects of the team's design on the work processes and subsequently on team performance are particularly evident when one examines the team's size. If the team is small but the best work procedures require a large team, the small size may prevent the team from using the most appropriate procedures for doing the work. Similarly, if the work requires that a wide variety of talent be applied to the work but the team is small, it may not have all the talent needed among its team members to accomplish the work (Cohen, 1994; Johnson & Johnson, 1994; Ray & Bronstein, 1995; Steiner, 1972).

Another example of the impacts of team design can be seen when one considers a team's goal clarity. Clear goals help the team identify the best procedures and resources to use and the knowledge and skill needed because it is clear what the end result is intended to be. Furthermore, unclear goals can negatively affect team effort because the time needed to discern the team's goals reduces the amount of time spent actually doing the work (Anderson & McDaniel, 1998; Barber & Iwai, 1996; Beyerlein & Johnson, 1994; Fisher, Rayner, & Belgard, 1995; Hitchcock & Willard, 1995; Ilgen & Klein, 1988; Johnson & Johnson, 1994; Landy & Becker, 1987; Locke & Latham, 1990; Manz & Sims, 1987; Plunkett & Fournier, 1991; Sims & Lorenzi, 1992; Zey, 1992).

Team Member Characteristics

The characteristics of team members have received less attention among theorists explaining EWT performance but appear to have important effects on the EWT's work process (Bielby & Bielby, 1989; Kettlitz, 1998; Lambert, 1990; Plunkett & Fournier, 1991; Robertson & Cummings, 1991; Steers & Spencer, 1977; Stewart, Carson, & Cardy, 1996; Williams & Alliger, 1994; Yeatts & Hyten, 1998). Team member characteristics include the team members' values, interests, needs, prejudices, supports outside work, and demographic characteristics such as education and age. Team member characteristics such as values, interests, prejudices, and needs can have direct effects on the work process, particularly the level of motivation and subsequently the amount of effort applied to the work. For example, an employee whose personal value system includes a belief that older people have gained many valuable experiences during their lives that are to be respected would be personally motivated in a job that entails providing care to older adults. On the other hand, if the person believes that older adults are outdated and have little value, then there is much less motivation to provide high-quality care.

SUMMARY AND CONCLUSION

With the growth of international competition, the manufacturing industry pushed to find better ways to use human resources. The result has been the establishment of nonmanagement work teams whose members are empowered to make decisions about their work such as scheduling the work, deciding who will do what on a particular day, and even identifying the training they need. These teams have proven to have high performance and low turnover if they are implemented successfully. Unfortunately, little scientific research has examined how these findings translate to human service organizations generally or to LTC organizations more specifically. However, it is clear that the lessons learned in manufacturing settings can only help those wanting to establish EWTs in LTC.

Factors that have been found to be most important to a team's success in non-LTC settings include the work process or how the work is actually accomplished (i.e., the knowledge and skill applied to the work, the procedures used, and the effort applied). Interpersonal processes have been found to be important to the work process factors. Effective communication, coordination, and cooperation improve the team's chances of using the most effective procedures and spending more time on the work itself, as opposed to discussing the work, arguing about how to do the work, and so on. Important environmental factors include management support, the reward system, training, and the culture of the organization. Important team design factors include the size of the team, clarity of goals, and procedures used to make decisions. Important team member characteristics include the values, interests, needs, and prejudices of the team members and the knowledge and skill they bring to the team.

CHAPTER 2

The Role of Empowered
Work Teams in Nursing Homes

In earlier centuries, older adults who had no family and no financial means to care for them spent their final years in poor houses, which were precursors to the earliest public hospitals. Nursing homes spun off from these hospitals, retaining essentially the same medical hierarchy of hospitals. The organizational management that results from this hierarchy leaves the people who spend the most time with and who provide the most direct care to nursing home residents with the least input into how this care will be provided. The introduction of empowered work teams (EWTs) into this equation offers an alternative management approach that capitalizes on the knowledge base and personal resources of this heretofore untapped part of the long-term care (LTC) workforce. This chapter describes what EWTs are and what role they can play in nursing homes.

It is helpful to begin with an understanding of the growth of the nursing home (NH) industry and how NHs have come to be organized. This is followed by a description of how NHs are staffed and organized and a discussion of the purposes and advantages of using EWTs in NHs. Next is a brief discussion of the types of EWTs that might be created, such as a direct care worker team, food service team, or housekeeping team. This is followed by a review of how an EWT might be designed, including goals and responsibilities, whom to include on the team, the size of the team, and use of team meetings, team notebooks, and team facilitators. Finally, a discussion of major factors affecting EWT performance in NHs is provided, including management support, decision-making methods and processes, and interpersonal processes.

GROWTH OF THE NURSING HOME INDUSTRY

At the turn of the 20th century most NHs were private, profit-making facilities that provided housing and medical care for those who could afford them. The only exceptions appear to have been some nonprofit facilities owned by religious or fraternal organizations. By the 1940s some states had begun to provide funds for the medical care of older adults, and in 1950 amendments to the Social Security Act permitted some funding for NH care of older adults. Also, during this time the Hill–Burton Act (1956) authorized federal funds for the construction of nonprofit NHs, and the Federal Housing Administration offered federally insured loans for the construction of for-profit NHs.

In 1960 Congress passed the Kerr–Mills Act, which allowed federal funds to be used to support some NH care for those who could not afford it. However, it was the enactment of the Medicaid program in 1965 that resulted in rapid growth of NHs. The Medicaid program was designed as a health insurance program for the poor, including coverage of skilled NH care if needed. This resulted in a tremendous growth in NHs, with many of them receiving a substantial portion of their revenue from Medicaid. Also, during this time the deinstitutionalization of residents in mental hospitals further increased the demand for NH care. As a result, the number of NH beds grew from 260,000 in 1954 to more than 1 million in the early 1970s. In 1999 there were 17,000 NHs supporting 1.6 million beds, and these numbers have continued to grow (Health Care Financing Administration, 2000; Quadagno, 2002; Uhlenberg, 1997).

STAFFING AND MANAGEMENT OF NURSING HOMES

The growth in the number of NH beds has brought about a growth in the size of NHs. As their size has increased, they have evolved to more bureaucratic or institutionalized health care. With larger size come the economic advantages of increasing efficiency by implementing bureaucratic rules and practices and increasing staff-to-patient ratios. As Thomas (2003, p. 149) notes,

> The skilled nursing facility's concentration of expertise, labor, equipment and elders has made sense for the same reason that a gigantic steel plant makes sense. These arrangements help the staff carry out necessary tasks in the quickest, most efficient manner possible. Greater operational efficiency opens the door to improved financial performance. Economic imperatives and the needs of professionals, not the desires of elders, have fostered largeness in long-term care.

Large NH size has facilitated a standardization of service by which all residents are expected to follow the same procedures. Consequently, the residents' personal preferences generally are not accommodated. For example, residents are often told when to wake up in the morning, eat meals, shower, and so on.

While the growth in NHs has spurred an emphasis on institutionalization, the medical profession has maintained a strict pecking order or hierarchy. Physicians are at the top and give the orders, and direct care workers are at the bottom and do what they are told. This has furthered the creation of a work environment that lacks warmth and friendliness, in which rules are not meant to be broken and participation in decision making by nonmanagement employees has not been an option.

Furthermore, the medical profession has implemented a medical model of care in the NH. Residents' physical health has been given the utmost priority. Although at face value this appears to be appropriate, the life satisfaction and preferences of the residents sometimes are overlooked or ignored (Weiner & Ronch, 2003). Evidence of the medical model in practice is apparent when those living in the nursing home are called "patients" and treated impersonally rather than "residents" living in their own home.

PURPOSE AND ADVANTAGES OF
EMPOWERED WORK TEAMS IN NURSING HOMES

Many providers of NH care are shifting their focus from a medical model of care to a person-centered model. This change in focus is the result of a desire among managers to make the NH a more enjoyable place to live and a more attractive alternative for those seeking NH care (Kane, 2001; Kane et al., 1997). NH providers who are successful at implementing this culture change are likely to have more and happier residents.

One component of the culture change, which has been encouraged by a variety of new NH initiatives, is the empowerment of direct care workers (e.g., certified nursing assistants, medical aides, restorative aides). A recent longitudinal study examining the effects of empowered direct care workers has found that EWTs result in improved direct care worker performance (see Chapter 6). Communication, cooperation, and information sharing within the NH improved, and family members gave them higher evaluation scores with regard to the staff listening, talking to and caring about the residents, checking on their comfort, spending time with them, and allowing them to choose when to eat and when to shower. Qualitative analyses found that the EWTs improved interpersonal processes that resulted in more informed direct care workers who were able to provide more personalized care to residents.

Empirical analyses have also found that when direct care workers are empowered, there are positive effects on job attitudes, such as job satisfaction and commitment, and negative effects on turnover and intent to quit. Qualitative analyses have found similar associations, including positive effects on direct care worker performance and reduced turnover as the direct care workers enjoyed their work more, felt less job burnout, and were more committed to the NH (see Chapters 5–7).

Although many positive effects have been found, the data also show that the positive effects are contingent on the successful implementation of the teams. These findings are no different from those found decades earlier in manufacturing settings. Poor implementation may result from such factors as a lack of involvement by nurse management, lack of effective facilitation of the team, insufficient time for team meetings, conflicts with the day or time of the weekly team meetings, or interpersonal conflicts within the team. When teams are not implemented appropriately they can have only minor positive effects, no effects, or even negative effects. Part III and the Appendix describe how to implement EWTs successfully.

TYPES OF EMPOWERED WORK TEAMS IN NURSING HOMES

Current experience with EWTs in NHs has been primarily with the establishment and monitoring of direct care worker EWTs. Therefore, this chapter focuses primarily on this group of NH employees. However, an NH may choose to establish EWTs among other groups of employees. The housekeeping staff is an ideal group to organize into EWTs. Most of these employees have the same or similar job titles, they have job responsibilities that are interchangeable, and they have the most direct knowledge about how best to perform the day-to-day tasks required. Food service staff also appear to be well suited to EWTs for the same reasons. Furthermore, the organization of the nursing staff into EWTs could bring many benefits, such as better communication among the nursing staff and routine discussions of processes that could be improved. Although nurses often meet together as a routine procedure in the nursing home, these meetings typically are held with the director of nursing present. An EWT made up of nurses would not include the director of nursing or assistant director of nursing. This would allow the nurses to discuss issues among themselves without the fear of retribution that can exist when a superior is at a meeting.

The establishment of EWTs among differing groups of employees can offer benefits beyond those specific to the teams and team members. EWTs of differing types can communicate with one another on a regular basis, provide each other with valuable information, and support one another. For example, housekeeping EWTs can enable housekeeping staff to communicate routinely with direct care workers. Housekeeping staff often have important information that they can share, ranging from observations about resident health conditions to housekeeping problems that warrant direct care worker assistance. A direct care worker EWT could benefit from regular communication with not only housekeeping EWTs but also food service EWTs (e.g., to congratulate a food service EWT for their promptness in delivering food or to request changes in the food delivery procedures).

Of course, such teams also provide opportunities for one group of employees to become overly critical of another. However, getting disagreements into the open allows all involved to become more informed about the issues and to reach understandings about problems that might otherwise continue to fester and reduce the quality of care provided.

DESIGN OF EMPOWERED WORK TEAMS IN NHS

The design of the EWT includes attention to the goals and responsibilities of the team, team composition, team size, the team facilitator, the team leader, and regular communications with management. Details on how to implement EWTs are provided in Part III; the focus in this chapter is on direct care worker EWTs.

Goals and Responsibilities of the Empowered Work Team

The goals and responsibilities of EWTs can range from those that allow high levels of empowerment and decision making regarding direct care workers to those that allow for little. Research suggests that it is best to design the EWT so that the level of empowerment is modest at first and increases as the team demonstrates an ability to accomplish assigned tasks and responsibilities. Furthermore, nurse management must be comfortable with the teams' goals and responsibilities. Some nurse managers have a management style that lends itself to empowerment, whereas others are less comfortable bringing others into the decision-making process. It is important that the specific nurse managers involved be comfortable with the goals and responsibilities being given to the EWTs. Just as important is the need to ensure that the direct care workers are adequately trained to accomplish the goals and responsibilities assigned to them. Numerous research studies have reported cases in which the members of EWTs were not adequately trained to take on their new responsibilities.

Goals assigned to EWTs might include developing recommendations for improving resident health and satisfaction, improving direct care work processes, and improving the work conditions of direct care workers (Exhibit 2A). How these are accomplished can vary greatly depending on the level of empowerment of the EWT. For example, when considering resident health and satisfaction, the EWT could meet weekly with nurse management and report on any resident conditions that they deem important. And a more empowered approach would be to ask the direct care workers to review resident health and satisfaction during their own weekly team meetings and then provide a summary of the meeting to nurse management. In this case, the direct care workers might review the cases of residents who appear to have emerging health problems or have problems that have not been addressed adequately. The results from this review would be recorded in a team notebook and provided to the nurse management. Added benefits of the latter approach are that (1) it gives direct care workers time to share information on the particular needs of specific residents; (2) if resident assignments change, all direct care workers would be prepared to provide the care these residents need; and

EXHIBIT 2A.
Purposes of Direct Care Worker Team Meetings

- To provide time during the week for direct care workers to discuss specific residents. For example, a direct care worker may want to talk about a resident who has been showing signs of having had a minor stroke or a resident who is having increasing problems with eating or controlling body functions.

- To allow direct care workers to respond to nurse management requests for ways to improve work processes. This can range from how to pass out meal trays so everyone gets a hot meal to how to respond to call lights in a timely fashion.

- To provide time for direct care workers to discuss personal issues. For example, a direct care worker might feel that she has been slighted by another or might not understand why a particular person is doing certain things. Team meetings enable direct care workers to discuss such things among themselves.

- To allow direct care workers to make recommendations to nurse management about how they might improve care and service to residents or improve aspects of their job.

- To allow nurse managers to comment on things that need to be improved or pass on compliments to direct care workers.

(3) direct care workers would better understand the work load of other direct care workers on their team and subsequently would be more open to offering help to those experiencing unusually heavy work loads.

A second goal that might be given to EWTs is to look for ways of improving the direct care work processes. The direct care workers know better than anyone else what works and what does not. They are the ones who actually carry out the work and are most aware of how easy or difficult it is to accomplish. Therefore, involving the EWT in developing or improving work processes can result in the use of processes that work better. Furthermore, studies have shown that when employees are involved in the development of a particular work process, they are more motivated to see that it is carried out. This goal can be accomplished by nurse management asking the EWTs to examine a particular work process and recommend ways for improving it. Nurse management may choose the particular work processes that are not working, that have received some complaints, or that have been noted for deficiencies. The direct care workers would then discuss the work process during weekly meetings and subsequently make a recommendation. Nurse management may then have the recommendation implemented or point out any parts of the recommendation that do not appear feasible and ask the team to revise their recommendation as needed. Once the recommendation is acceptable to both nurse management and the EWT, it is implemented.

A third goal of EWTs might be to help nurse management create a work environment that is inviting to direct care workers. The EWT can be consulted on issues ranging from how and when to assign work breaks to the type of sanitary gloves the direct care workers prefer. It is important that management not ask for advice from the EWTs unless they are genuinely open to implementing their suggestions.

People Included in an Empowered Work Team

By definition, EWTs are made up of employees who are of similar job title or rank. It is important that they be similar in rank so that they feel free to give their opinions without concern that a superior will reprimand them. Furthermore, an advantage of having the same job title is that they can focus on issues of mutual concern. For example, an EWT of direct care workers might discuss how to best deliver meals to residents, whereas a housekeeping EWT might discuss the best time for and approach to changing residents' bed sheets.

An EWT often includes members who work on the same shift and serve the same residents. For example, an NH with 50 residents might have one EWT of direct care workers who work the day shift and are responsible for all the residents in the NH. An evening EWT would be responsible for all the residents during the evening shift. For a much larger NH, there might be several day shift EWTs, with each serving its own wings, floors, or halls of the NH and, likewise, several evening shift EWTs, with each EWT serving the residents in specific areas of the NH. Some NHs have separate staff who work on the weekends, in which case they would establish EWTs made up of the direct care workers who work only on the weekends.

In determining who should participate on a particular team, it can be valuable to include people from different shifts who serve the same residents. One advantage to a multishift team is that the employees on the two shifts can review residents during their team meeting and get a fuller picture of the residents' daily activities, eating habits, and so on. Another advantage is that the employees can discuss issues surrounding the shift change and any concerns that the employees of one shift have about the performance of those on the other. A disadvantage of this approach is that many work processes are unique to one shift, so that when the process is being discussed during a team meeting, those on the other shift might have no input or involvement. For example, the direct care workers on the day shift may want to discuss the procedures used for preparing residents for breakfast. The direct care workers on the evening shift might want to discuss the procedures for preparing residents for bed. Neither group is involved with the other's procedures and so will be left out of discussions. An alternative is to have two teams, one for the day shift and one for the evening shift, and to have one person who participates in the meetings of both teams, or the members of each team might take turns participating in both teams' meetings. This allows communication and information sharing between the shifts without the disadvantages noted here.

Creating direct care worker EWTs that work the night shift has been found to be difficult. Often the NH has only a small number of direct care workers working during this time, and those who are working often are caring for different groups of residents. Furthermore, of these direct care workers, some do not work regularly on the night shift. Instead, they regularly work on the day or evening shifts and choose to work occasionally on the night shift for additional pay. The combination of a small number of regular direct care workers, those who do not serve the same group of residents, and the lack of continuity in who works at night makes it difficult to create night shift EWTs.

Size of the Empowered Work Team

The optimal size for an EWT depends largely on the particular area of the NH that the team is serving and, more specifically, the number of residents being served and the amount of care these residents need. The number of team members should reflect the number of direct care workers needed to adequately serve the residents living in the team's target area. Given these constraints on team size, research suggests that the ideal size of an EWT is four to seven members (Brightman, 1988; Ray & Bronstein, 1995). It has been found that this size allows all team members to participate in discussions and provide input during decision making. This has the benefit of using the knowledge of all the direct care workers on the team and creating a situation in which all team members feel a responsibility to carry out the decisions made and a responsibility to their teammates.

When the team reaches a size of 10 or more, some direct care workers do not participate in the meetings, often are not engaged or aware of the topics being discussed, and simply wait for the others to make decisions. It has also been found that a large team is more likely to result in a few team members dominating the decision-making process and those less involved feeling no responsibility to carry out the decisions made and feeling no responsibility to the others on the team. Furthermore, a large team can divide into factions that routinely disagree with one another.

Means of Carrying Out Team Goals: Empowered Work Team Meetings

Direct care worker EWTs typically hold at least one 30-minute sit-down meeting a week. The direct care workers choose a day and time to meet that they feel is best for them (e.g., a slow time during their work shift). Ideally, all team members who are on duty attend the meeting. While the team is meeting, the nurses on duty assist the team by performing direct care worker duties (e.g., answering call lights).

Each team has a team leader or coordinator and a backup team leader or coordinator. These people are responsible for making sure the team meets each week, that the team meetings focus on the team agenda or what needs to be covered, and that everyone on the team has an opportunity to share their views during the meeting. The person serving as the team leader or coordinator typically is selected by the team but, if deemed necessary, can be assigned by nurse management.

The agenda for the team meeting should reflect the goals of the team. Exhibit 11A in Chapter 11 provides a list of topics that a team might address. One approach found to be successful is for a list of topics to be included in a team notebook and for the team to review the list each week. For example, the team might begin the meeting by addressing the following questions:

- Are there any issues or procedures related to our work that we should discuss today?

- Has the nursing staff given our team any problems to work on this week?

  Other typical questions include the following:

- Have any of the residents on your hall developed a skin problem or stopped eating? What are you doing to help them with these problems? Any recommendations?

- Have any residents displayed behavioral problems that are different from what they normally display? What are you doing, if anything, to resolve these problems?

- Has anyone completed an incident report recently? If so, please tell us what happened.

Training should be provided to team members to assist them in the decision-making process. Such training becomes particularly valuable when the team is addressing a problem that has multiple solutions and the team is attempting to determine which is best.

In addition to a weekly sit-down meeting, the EWT has brief stand-up meetings as needed throughout the week. The purpose of these meetings is to address concerns that need immediate attention. For example, if it is learned that a team member is going to be absent from work unexpectedly, the team can hold a brief stand-up meeting to decide how the work will be reassigned until a replacement direct care worker arrives. In some cases, a stand-up meeting will allow the team to arrive at a temporary solution to a problem, such as a resident complaint, until the team has time to examine the problem more thoroughly and arrive at a more permanent solution.

Means of Carrying Out Team Goals: The Team Notebook

Each EWT has a team folder or three-ring notebook. The notebook contains a weekly sign-in sheet for those attending the meeting, a topic sheet or agenda providing various questions that the team might want to address during the meeting, sheets for taking weekly notes of the meetings, a decision guide sheet to assist team members during the decision-making process, and sheets for nurse management to communicate to the teams. During weekly meetings, someone on the team other than the team leader volunteers to take notes for that week (team training sessions should emphasize that perfect spelling is not necessary for taking notes). All major issues discussed during the meeting are noted. Examples of major issues include a health-related issue of a specific resident, a broken shower head that is still not working correctly, and complaints of verbal abuse from a specific nurse. Team notes are read weekly by nurse management, which may include the director of nursing and the EWT's immediate supervisor. Nurse management then provides feedback to the team, by writing a response and including it in the team's notebook to be read at the next meeting or calling for a brief stand-up meeting to address the issue more immediately. Nurse management may also use this feedback format to request that the team recommend a suggestion or solution for a particular problem, although it is recommended that the problem be presented to the team in person so that any questions can be answered immediately.

Means of Carrying Out Team Goals: The Team Facilitator

New EWTs typically need a team facilitator. This is a nonthreatening person who can help the team get together once a week, review their agenda items, work through the decision-making process, make sure that someone takes notes during the meetings, and make sure that nurse management reads the notes and responds to the team each week. This might include an employee from the NH's personnel office, someone from another non-nursing position, or perhaps a medical or restorative aide who has earned the respect of the direct care workers but is not a supervisor of them. The team facilitator receives training in how best to assist the team (see the Appendix for facilitator training guidelines). As the team members gain confidence in their new role as EWT members, the facilitator can occasionally skip a team meeting and eventually attend meetings infrequently.

FACTORS AFFECTING EMPOWERED WORK TEAM PERFORMANCE IN NURSING HOMES

Many factors affect EWT performance (Becker-Reems, 1994; Campion, Medsker, & Higgs, 1993; Cohen, 1994; Neuhaus, 1990; Tannenbaum, Beard, & Salas, 1992; Yeatts & Hyten, 1998). Three factors are of particular importance for EWTs in NHs: management support, decision-making methods and processes, and interpersonal processes.

Management Support

Previous research has found that management support is crucial to the success of empowered work teams (Sims & Lorenzi, 1992; Yeatts & Hyten, 1998). In the NH setting, perhaps the single most important form of support is to provide the EWTs with an opportunity to have input into decisions related to their day-to-day tasks. In many cases, this might mean that nurse management makes a temporary decision, such as a new procedure for direct care workers to answer call lights, and requests that the EWTs develop a permanent solution. In such cases, it is important that nurse management provide the EWTs with all the information they need to develop an effective solution. For example, in the case of call lights, such information should include the reasons why a new method is being sought (e.g., complaints from residents or family members) and a description of the specific problems with the previous procedures. It is also important that nurse management not already have a "best" procedure in mind, with the idea that they will continue to have the team work on the issue until the team itself suggests this "best" procedure. Supportive nurse management will be willing to try the recommendations of the EWT unless it is clear that they might be harmful. In these cases, a complete explanation for why the solution is inappropriate should be provided to the team and the team given an opportunity to revise their solution. Otherwise, the team should be given the opportunity to try their solution and learn from their mistakes.

Another means of providing support is to faithfully read and respond to any EWT questions or comments provided in weekly team notes. This means that nurse management must set aside time each week to review these notes. If nurse management is not routinely reading and responding to the team notes, then the direct care workers begin to wonder why they should bother meeting because their thoughts and concerns are not being heard and their recommendations are being ignored. On the other hand, if the direct care workers believe that nurse management truly cares what they think and respects their opinions, as evidenced by nurse management's responses to the meeting notes, they will respond more positively to the daily comments and requests from nurse management.

Still other ways of providing support include helping out when the direct care workers are in their team meetings or when the direct care workers are short staffed or otherwise overloaded with work and providing positive reinforcement when the EWT is successful. A nurse who is willing to do "direct care work" when help is needed gains respect from direct care workers, who subsequently become more open to the nurse's suggestions and requests. Positive reinforcement can be as simple as a "good job" comment in the EWT notebook or more substantial reinforcements such as gift certificates for the team. Positive reinforcement can encourage the direct care workers to continue trying and provides them with guidelines for high performance.

Decision-Making Methods and Processes

A decision-making *method* is a sequence of steps that a team follows before making a decision. The decision-making *process* is the means by which the team selects a choice once the decision-making method has been completed, such as the use of consensus and majority vote. EWTs with little empowerment have almost no decision-making authority at the team level; instead, decisions are made by the nurse. As EWTs gain experience and training and are given the opportunity to make decisions, they typically follow a sequence of steps, including considering several alternatives, weighing the pros and cons of each, and selecting the best one (see Chapter 11). It is extremely helpful when those on the team have a high level of respect for one another and one another's viewpoints. It is important that they listen to one another and not be afraid to disagree when they have a different view.

One issue of concern is the time-consuming nature of decision making. However, it has been found that in stand-up meetings, EWTs can make decisions effectively in a short time. For example, when deciding how to address a desire or need of a resident, direct care workers typically have a stand-up meeting in which they clarify the issue, consider the pros and cons of various alternatives, and then select a solution, all within roughly 5 minutes. If more time is needed, the team members can defer making a decision until more time can be applied to the problem (e.g., during a slower part of the work day).

The decision-making process often used by EWTs is consensus, that is, making a team decision that all team members are willing to support and no team member opposes (Yeatts & Hyten, 1998). When consensus cannot be reached, the nurse supervisor or nurse management might be asked to help the team achieve consensus; failing this, the team might need to go with the majority opinion. If time allows, the team can set the issue aside temporarily, rather than making a decision that some team members disagree with, and then revisit it after all team members have had an opportunity to think more about it. One shortcoming of this approach is the possibility that a decision is never reached, and the problem persists.

Interpersonal Processes

Much of the research on work teams has focused on the interpersonal processes within the team (Holt, 1990; Johnson & Johnson, 1994; McGrath, 1964). These include processes such as communication, coordination, cooperative conflict, and trust. Generally, these improve as team members are given the opportunity to practice them in their team meetings. As these skills develop, they have positive effects, not only during the team meetings but also throughout the work day. And these improved interpersonal skills are applied not only to other direct care workers but also to nurse management, food staff, custodial staff, residents, and residents' families and friends.

Developing interpersonal skills is not easy, and individuals must have opportunities to practice the skills. EWT meetings provide such opportunities. A team facilitator can help team members recognize when they are demonstrating a lack of skill. As direct care workers communicate regularly with one another in the team meetings, their skills can improve and trust can develop. It is not uncommon for direct care workers who have not spoken or assisted one another for weeks or months to change this behavior once they begin meeting as a team and work through their differences. This also builds trust between team members. EWT members begin to believe that others on the team will look out for their welfare and assist them in times of need. Team members begin to seek out and value the approval of one another and attempt to earn it by performing high-quality work and assisting others on the team.

One example of such interpersonal skill development was observed when an EWT was first created. A short time after the team meeting began, it became clear that two team members were not speaking to one another or assisting one another during the day. As the meeting progressed, one of the two direct care workers brought up the importance of trust between team members. The discussion quickly led to an accusation by one of the direct care workers that the other had given false information to their supervisor about her work performance. A heated discussion ensued in which the accused direct care worker denied the accusations and suggested that perhaps the supervisor got false information through another means. The result of this heated discussion was that the two direct care workers apologized to one another. This spilled over to the work environment, where they no longer attempted to avoid one another and began offering help to one another. Trust grew between the two, and the NH residents benefited from the improved care they received.

CONCLUSION

EWTs in NHs can be made up of direct care workers, housekeepers, food service staff, and nurses. Their level of empowerment can range from a great deal of decision-making responsibility to very little. Their purpose is to improve resident care while making the work more enjoyable. EWTs carry out their decision-making responsibilities through both impromptu stand-up meetings and weekly scheduled sit-down meetings that include reviewing an agenda of topics (see Chapter 11, Exhibit 11A) and taking weekly minutes of their meetings. Effectiveness of the EWTs relies heavily on management support, proper EWT decision-making procedures, and sensitive interpersonal processes. The EWTs' efforts can have positive effects on staff attitudes, resident care, and family member perceptions of care.

CHAPTER 3

The Potential for Empowered Work Teams in Assisted Living Communities

Mauro Hernandez

Assisted living (AL) is one of several terms used to describe non–nursing home, residential settings. AL communities differ in the amount of service available, the residential character of the environment, and the support for consumer values of privacy, independence, and choice (Kane & Wilson, 2001). Like other long-term care (LTC) provider categories, AL settings have experienced high levels of turnover, particularly among staff who provide the majority of direct care services and work most closely with residents. Reported turnover rates among direct care workers in AL range from about 40% to more than 100%—lower than in nursing homes but higher than in home health agencies (Wright, 2005).

As one of the fastest-growing sectors in the aging services field, AL providers face increasing challenges in recruiting and retaining qualified workers. Such challenges are linked to increases in the size of the older population, projected workforce shortages, and increased competition from other AL facilities and home- and community-based service providers. Government projections based on future demand for LTC services show that the number of direct care workers employed in residential care settings will need to increase by 67%, from about 311,000 in 2000 to about 518,000 in 2010 (Department of Health and Human Services et al., 2003). However, direct care work in AL is characterized by low wages and benefits, limited training, and high injury rates (Wright, 2005). Therefore, AL providers must continue to explore alternative management practices that help increase and improve their workforce.

This chapter considers the potential application of empowered work teams (EWTs) in AL settings. First, AL is defined within the LTC continuum, with a focus on how this sector has grown and evolved in the 1980s, 1990s, and early 21st century. This is followed by a discussion of the different management and staffing arrangements found in AL, based on prior research and firsthand experience in the field. Finally, this chapter discusses some of the key characteristics and practices of EWTs and how they might be applied in AL settings.

SITUATING ASSISTED LIVING IN THE LONG-TERM CARE FIELD

The broad term *assisted living* is used to describe a range of supportive housing options that are generally licensed under a variety of names. Although various stakeholders disagree about how AL should be defined, there is consensus that AL organizations include non–nursing home, residential settings that provide or arrange room, board, personal care, health-related services, and 24-hour oversight.

AL often is conceptualized on a continuum or array of LTC options. Nursing homes occupy the highest position on such a continuum by providing a range of LTC options with high service capacity and cost. At the other end are services provided by individuals and organizations to clients living in their own homes. The broad category of AL settings, which includes traditional residential care, often is conceived as falling somewhere in the middle, depending on working definitions and the criteria being used to examine building and service characteristics. When the last nationally representative study was conducted in 1998, the typical AL setting was a freestanding organization operating for less than 10 years and licensed to provide personal assistance to about 50 residents (Hawes, Rose, & Phillips, 1999). Other studies have also included smaller settings (5–10 residents) that may represent a very large proportion of a state's AL bed supply (Hedrick et al., 2003; Newcomer, Breuer, & Zhang, 1994; Salmon, Hyer, Hedgecock, Zayac, & Engh, 2004).

The precursor to AL was "mom-and-pop" operations. Known as boarding homes or board and care homes, these small settings provided personal care and oversight for a handful of clients, often in the service provider's own home (Pratt, 2004). Starting in the late 1800s, "homes for the aged" were established as a larger and related type of facility, often owned and operated by state or county governments to meet the housing and care needs of indigent people. More recent forms of group residential care include campus-style continuing care retirement communities, smaller adult foster homes, and larger adult congregate housing with coordinated services (Kane & Wilson, 1993).

A newer form of residential care called assisted living emerged in the mid- to late 1980s, initially attempting to distinguish itself from traditional board and care. AL often is described as a more market-driven model that grew in response to the availability of private development financing, state LTC policy developments, and consumer preferences (Hawes et al., 1999; Wilson, 1995). Entrepreneurial efforts in different parts of the country developed hybrid settings that looked more like traditional single-family homes and had a higher service capacity than traditional board and care, thus allowing residents to age in place (Wilson, in press). These newer settings also tended to target a more affluent population, except in a few states whose Medicaid policies motivated AL communities to serve low-income residents. Early projects typically were financed through some combination of owner equity, private investor groups, and small business loans.

State agencies also began to change their residential care programs in response to local market activity, quality of care issues, and state fiscal concerns. A growing supply of AL settings began serving residents whose needs often conflicted with outdated licensing regulations yet who were similar to the increasingly dependent home care recipients. Government reports pointed to uneven state regulatory oversight and resident care problems (GAO, 1989, 1992). At the same time, other reports provided evidence that states could reduce nursing home use and related Medicaid expenditures by adopting policies that included increasing the supply and facilitating access to less costly AL services by Medicaid nursing home–eligible residents (Alecxih, Lutzky, Corea, & Coleman, 1996; Doty, 2000; Wiener & Stevenson, 1998). As a result, state regulatory and financing policies have changed in varying degrees to allow AL communities to serve more impaired, lower-income residents under increasingly specific conditions (Mollica & Johnson-Lamarche, 2005).

Recent Growth Factors

The AL industry has experienced rapid growth, particularly in the 1990s. From 1990 to 2002, the number of licensed AL communities increased by more than half, and bed supply almost doubled (Harrington, Chapman, Miller, Miller, & Newcomer, 2005). However, there has been wide variation across states in terms of AL bed supply and growth rates in recent years, partly because of state policies and economic developments. By 2004, Oregon had the largest AL bed supply, with 64 beds per 1,000 older adults (age 65 and up), followed by Maine, Virginia, California, and Pennsylvania. By comparison, the lowest-ranked states—Louisiana, Illinois, Mississippi, Iowa, and Arkansas—had between 8 and 12 beds per 1,000 older adults (Newcomer, Flores, & Hernandez, in press).

A variety of AL forms have emerged, whether shaped by state policies or market forces. Overall growth has been fueled largely by private rather than public financing and payment sources. Compared with growth in the nursing home sector, which was fueled largely by public development financing and reimbursement, growth in AL facilities has depended much less on state and federal funding. Private financing options for new AL ventures expanded rapidly in the 1990s as developers secured capital through public offerings on Wall Street, larger commercial loans, real estate investment trusts, and venture capital (Nordheimer, 1995; Pallarito, 1995). Even in a year of declining Wall Street financing, there were 15 public offerings in 1997, worth a total of $1.4 billion, and another $12.4 billion in private capital was available to support continued AL growth (Vickery, 1998). These sources of capital fueled regional and national expansion efforts for newly established AL chains (e.g., Assisted Living Concepts and Sunrise). Diversification efforts by other large organizations with origins in hospitality management (e.g., Hyatt and Marriott), nursing homes (e.g., Beverly Enterprises and Manor Care), and senior housing (e.g., American Retirement and Holiday Retirement) may have also stimulated AL growth (Nordheimer, 1995). Furthermore, it is likely that smaller operators benefited indirectly from these developments as AL came to be viewed as a less risky and more legitimate investment opportunity among conventional lenders and private investors.

Organizational Forms

The AL industry consists of multiple organizational forms, such as a "housing with services" model that is geared more toward housekeeping and social services than personal care, a "personal care" model resembling traditional board and care, and a more service-intensive "nursing home replacement" (or aging in place) model designed to provide an intermediate level of care (Wilson, 1994). Recent studies differentiate AL forms by service capacity and physical environment characteristics. For example, Hawes and colleagues (1999) use five classifications to categorize the national AL supply based on reported levels of service (high or low) and privacy (high, low, or minimal). Those categorized as offering high levels of service and privacy represent a small proportion (11%) of AL organizations in the United States. A variety of other classification strategies, whether distinguished by size, licensing category, age, or services, have been used to describe organizational characteristics within and between states and have been linked with resident characteristics and outcomes (Hedrick et al., 2003; Newcomer et al., 1994; Salmon et al., 2004; Zimmerman et al., 2003).

AL organizations vary in terms of the types of services they are willing or able to provide. Core services typically include some level of personal care assistance, medication supervision, social and recreational activities, meals, and housekeeping. What seems to distinguish organizations is the intensity of personal care assistance an organization provides and the availability of other specialized healthcare and behavioral services (Hernandez, 2006). Consequently, AL forms have emerged that serve different segments of the LTC population, ranging from those who need minimal assistance with activities of daily living (ADLs) to those who would otherwise be in a nursing facility because of intermittent nursing needs, dependence in ADLs, or advanced cognitive and behavioral limitations (Hawes et al., 1999; Zimmerman, Sloane, & Eckert, 2001).

Other aspects of an organization's residency criteria and price may further segment the targeted market by resident payment source and income. Nationally, only 18% of administrators interviewed from high-privacy, high-service AL communities have reported having at least one publicly subsidized resident. A small proportion of AL administrators accept Supplemental Security Income (18%) or Medicaid (11%), and almost half (45%) discharge residents when they exhaust their private funds (Hawes, Phillips, & Rose, 2000). Pricing policies vary by type of organization, available services, resident unit amenities, and geographic market (Hawes et al., 2000; MetLife, 2005; Wylde, 1998). Findings suggest that AL services may be priced higher than what typical LTC users are able to afford (Hawes et al., 2000; Wylde, 1998).

Wide variation in physical environmental characteristics also has been reported between and within states. AL types may be distinguished by the number of residents typically permitted in each unit or sleeping area, the type of personal living space available, and the total number of people served (Han, Sirrocco, & Rembsburg, 2003). For example, one type includes adapted single-family homes or purpose-built structures designed to accommodate a handful of people in shared- or private-bedroom units. Owners typically are the primary caregivers, with additional staff hired depending on resident needs, state requirements, and size (Carder, Morgan, & Eckert, 2005). In terms of overall bed supply, estimates from national and multistate studies suggest that the most common AL settings are those that serve about 50 residents who live in private or semiprivate rooms (Hawes et al.,

1999; Zimmerman et al., 2003). These include newer purpose-built facilities, older board and care homes, and, to a lesser extent, converted nursing home wings. A third, more recently developed AL type is distinguished by providing individual living units that contain features typically found in an apartment, such as full private bathrooms and kitchenettes.

MANAGEMENT AND STAFFING ARRANGEMENTS IN ASSISTED LIVING

When examining staffing in AL settings, most studies and policy reports focus on staffing levels, qualifications, and training. These are largely descriptive studies that examine how such factors vary by state licensing requirements and across facility types. Little attention has been given to how AL staff are involved in service planning, scheduling, and team coordination efforts. This section describes AL employees and how they are typically organized, as reported in selected studies and observed in the author's field experiences and communications with other practitioners.

Staffing Features Across Settings and Models

Regardless of size, licensed AL organizations employ an administrator or executive director to oversee daily operations in accordance with state regulations. Requirements for AL administrators vary by state and by organizational practice. For example, in some states a person with a high school degree and some related direct care or management experience might be permitted to operate an AL community after having completed a training course. In other states, a qualified administrator might need a bachelor's degree in a related health or social service field, a nursing home or AL administrator license, or one or more years of experience in a related setting (National Center for Assisted Living, 2007).

The staffing arrangements found in AL organizations are highly influenced by the experience, education, and training of the AL administrator. This is to be expected because administrators draw on the knowledge and experiences gained from having worked in other settings. As a result, AL managers may organize staff and service delivery based on common organizational blueprints found in senior housing, skilled nursing facilities, hotels, hospitals, or home health agencies.

Moving down the organizational hierarchy, other supervisory and skilled staff may be found in larger AL communities where organizational structures resemble those of nursing facilities. In such settings, workers are organized into functional areas such as administration, dietary, housekeeping, maintenance, direct care, health-related services, marketing, and activity departments. Supervisors then coordinate, plan, and oversee the work performed in their respective departments. Nurses may also play key roles in organizing and coordinating direct care workers. However, AL providers differ in their use of licensed nurses, who may serve as administrators, care coordinators, caregivers, or consultants (Hawes, Phillips, Rose,

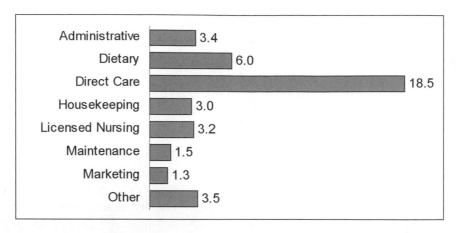

Administrative   3.4
Dietary   6.0
Direct Care   18.5
Housekeeping   3.0
Licensed Nursing 3.2
Maintenance   1.5
Marketing   1.3
Other   3.5

Figure 3.1. Full-Time Equivalent Staff by Department. *Note:* Estimates are based on a 50-unit AL facility using the mean full-time equivalent staff per 100 residents, as reported in *The 2006 Overview of Assisted Living* (2006).

Holan, & Sherman, 2003). An industry-sponsored study shows that the majority of AL staff are direct care workers, followed by dietary, administrative, licensed nursing, and housekeeping personnel (Figure 3.1).

One key feature that typically distinguishes AL from other unlicensed supportive housing settings is the availability of 24-hour direct care staff to provide oversight and meet residents' scheduled and unscheduled service needs. Beyond this, state and organizational policies differ in terms of required staffing levels and the qualifications and training required to provide personal care, dietary, and health-related services. Although few states require AL providers to have specific staff-to-resident ratios, most (86%) specify that there must be "sufficient staff" in numbers and qualifications to meet resident service needs (Mollica & Johnson-Lamarche, 2005).

Use of Universal Workers

A common practice in AL is the use of universal workers, who are cross-trained and responsible for providing personal care, medication, dining, housekeeping, and laundry services. According to Hawes and colleagues (2000), most staff who provide personal care services in high-service or high-privacy AL communities are also responsible for other tasks, such as meal preparation, housekeeping, and laundry. Findings from a more recent industry-sponsored survey suggest that freestanding AL communities may be more likely to adopt a universal worker approach to staffing than those that are affiliated with an independent living facility, nursing facility, or continuing care retirement community (*The 2006 Overview of Assisted Living*, 2006). State policies may also influence the use of universal workers. For example, licensing regulations and nurse practice requirements differ with respect to the provision of medication and health-related services by licensed nurses and unlicensed personnel (Reinhard, Young, Kane, & Quinn, 2006; Wagner, Nadash, & Sabatino, 1997). Although unlicensed workers may perform such tasks under a nurse's training and supervision in some states, only licensed nurses or specially certified workers can do so in other states. Other government restrictions may limit the scope of services that may be provided by caregivers employed as universal workers.

Furthermore, as organizations grow, work activities tend to become more specialized and functionally segmented. Services that might otherwise be provided by the same one or two caregivers in a very small community often are divided up in larger communities across staff who are specifically trained and responsible for providing only maintenance, laundry, housekeeping, personal care, marketing, dietary, recreational, or health-related services. In these more departmentalized AL settings, separate job descriptions designate people who are responsible for organizing a game of cards, applying skin lotion, hanging a picture, making a resident's bed, providing help with a shower, or serving a meal.

Although greater division of labor may be desirable in other settings where work involves fairly repetitive or highly skilled tasks, structuring AL services in this way may have unintended consequences. A common belief among managers is that greater efficiency, reliability, and accountability may be achieved by allocating work across such functionally specified roles. One assumption is that specialized knowledge and experience equip workers to deliver services more effectively and consistently in multiple situations. Creating distinct functional roles allows AL managers to assign tasks to specific people with the expectation that the work will be performed correctly. It also facilitates follow-up. Although this arrangement may reassure residents who expect service providers to be appropriately qualified, it may also lead to frustration or avoidable delays when service needs are less easily anticipated or scheduled. In AL settings where services are highly segmented, residents may be expected to direct different types of requests to the particular staff who are qualified or permitted to address them. A common example used to illustrate this problem is the housekeeper who is cleaning up a resident's apartment but is not qualified to help the resident use the bathroom. Regardless of how urgent the resident's need is, he or she must wait until an appropriately qualified worker arrives.

In the last decade, AL developers and operators have experimented with alternative structures and practices to ensure customer responsiveness and efficiency. One option that is more commonly found in less urban areas is to locate three or four smaller AL homes on the same or adjacent properties. Much like in the recently emerging Green House nursing home model (Kane, Lum, Cutler, Degenholtz, & Yu, 2007), individual AL homes may have between 5 and 20 residents and are staffed with a primary caregiver and designed with a small common kitchen and dining room. Administrative and intermittent skilled nursing oversight are shared across the multiple smaller homes (see chapter 5 for discussion of EWTs and the Green House concept). A parallel approach found in larger, urban AL settings involves designing or adapting facilities with self-contained clusters of rooms or floors that have their own dining and activity areas. Caregivers or universal workers are specifically assigned to the residents in their cluster, and other administrative, maintenance, and skilled nursing staff members have floating responsibilities for the whole facility. The most common example is found in AL communities with a designated wing or floor for residents who are more cognitively impaired. Such structures and practices have existed for several years, although little is known about the extent of their adoption, much less their costs or benefits.

EMPOWERING EMPLOYEES IN ASSISTED LIVING

It is reasonable to expect that AL providers will be receptive to the notion of adopting practices to empower their employees. Benefits could be expected in terms of improved worker performance and attitudes and reduced turnover rates. In general, AL providers have a shared interest in promoting residents' quality of life. Industry advocates often emphasize the more customer-oriented environments AL communities provide and the philosophical orientation that promotes resident privacy, independence, individuality, and choice in more homelike settings. Although such providers may be less constrained by formal structures, it is reasonable to expect that hierarchical management practices are common in AL settings, particularly in larger ones or those that are affiliated with other levels of care.

A push for less institutionalized and more individualized care across the LTC continuum is led by the Pioneer Network and its culture change movement. In discussing key elements of this culture change, Lustbader (2001) describes a range of strategies for nursing homes that could also be—and in some cases have been—adopted by AL managers to increase the capacity of workers to be more responsive to resident needs and preferences. First, the managers of larger AL communities might consider eliminating or restructuring middle layers of management and integrating departmental functions. Second, rather than using multiple supervisors to oversee functionally segmented departments directly, managers might organize direct care workers into EWTs and give them the authority to negotiate routine aspects of their work independently while consulting as needed with others who have specialized skills and knowledge. By combining the fairly well-recognized concept of universal workers with the cluster care arrangements noted previously, such facilities would take advantage of the universal workers' knowledge of the individual residents and provide a setting that has been found to improve job attitudes (see Chapter 8). Third, AL managers may more actively involve EWTs in the processes being used to review and modify individualized service plans. Often, staff input is limited to a manager's or service coordinator's review of documented service refusals, incident reports, and patterns of service use. A more involved approach would be to invite one or more team members from different shifts to attend meetings in which individual service plans are being reviewed.

Future work is needed that more directly examines current organizational structures and management practices in AL, with a focus on management practices that can empower universal workers. Although AL may be a less institutional arrangement than traditional nursing home care, increasing facility size and state regulatory requirements have resulted in hierarchical structures and departmentalized service delivery that do not take advantage of the knowledge and experience direct care workers can provide. Fortunately, smaller AL settings seem to be the wave of the future (Sikorska, 1999). These settings may be particularly conducive to an EWT made up of universal workers. Some larger AL providers have already restructured their staffing and service delivery systems to more closely resemble smaller homes that are part of a larger community. These are ripe for establishing EWTs that enable universal workers to use their knowledge and experience to make decisions that improve resident health and worker attitudes.

CHAPTER 4

The Potential for Empowered Work Teams in Home Care Settings

Katherina A. Nikzad, Keith A. Anderson, and Joseph E. Gaugler

Home health care encompasses a wide range of health and supportive services for people who are disabled, aging, and chronically ill and in need of treatment or functional assistance in the home. Also embedded in the home care philosophy is the goal of restoring the client to or maintaining the client at the highest possible level of health, functioning, and comfort in a familiar environment. Thus home care is appropriate in many instances, especially when a family member or friend cannot provide assistance on a consistent basis or when placement in a long-term facility is not feasible (Buhler-Wilkerson, 2001; Morris, Caro, & Hansan, 1998).

This chapter provides a discussion of the historical context of home care, including its evolution, its present state, and future trends. This is followed by an examination of the staffing patterns of home care organizations, including proprietary or for-profit agencies, not-for-profit agencies, government or official agencies, and health disciplines that are represented in home care. Finally, the use of empowered work teams (EWTs) and other innovations for providing home care service is considered.

HISTORICAL CONTEXT OF HOME CARE

Since its advent, home health care has undergone several transformations, based on different historical contexts and different motives for its inception. Examining the evolution of home care, including its origins and progression over time, provides a more refined understanding of how and why home care has become what it is today and how researchers and health care professionals should continue to evaluate and improve it.

Evolution of Home Care

Providing care for people in the home environment is not a novel concept. In fact, historical accounts reveal that home care was common among the families of people who experienced an array of health problems. The conception of home care can be traced back as early as the 1700s, when physicians made regular home visits. In 1796 a group of citizens in Boston, Massachusetts, formed the first permanent medical institution in New England, known as the Boston Dispensary. This institution provided free medical care to those who could not afford it. This innovation was a powerful force in American medical history because the dispensary was the first in the country to provide a visiting nurse association, dental clinic, rehabilitative clinic, and child services. The dispensary later merged with the Floating Hospital and Pratt Diagnostic Clinic in 1965 to form what is currently known as the New England Medical Center (Spiegel, 1987).

In the 1800s an important development in home care was the establishment of home nursing services. These consisted of laypeople providing skilled care to the ill and education to family members who provided a portion of the in-home care. Toward the end of the 1800s, a voluntary organization was established in New York to provide nursing care to people living at home. In the years that followed, several other voluntary organizations were initiated in Massachusetts and Pennsylvania, providing similar care to people living at home. These voluntary organizations later came to be known as visiting nurse associations (Buhler-Wilkerson, 2001; Spiegel, 1987).

Home Care in the 20th Century

In the mid-1900s it was common for people to receive a large portion of their medical care in the home rather than in a hospital. Receiving care in a hospital in the earlier part of this era often was viewed negatively because it was believed that people who entered hospitals rarely returned home. Receiving care in the home also became more feasible by the early 20th century because life insurance companies included home care as a benefit. By this time, visiting nurse services were expanding throughout the country, making it even more feasible for people to receive health care at home (Buhler-Wilkerson, 2001; Spiegel, 1987).

In tandem with the development and expansion of home care services, the United States also witnessed several important medical advancements in the 20th century. The development of antibiotics, immunizations, and improvements in nutrition and sanitation changed many diseases that were once considered deadly to long-term illnesses. Thus more people began living longer with their illnesses than in previous decades. This development had many implications for health care providers and ultimately led to an increase in the number of long-term care institutions and the establishment of the medical model as the prevailing ideology of chronic care (Peters & McKeon, 1998; Stein, 2001).

Institutional care dominated the health care system in the first half of the 20th century, but home care resurged in 1947 when Dr. E. M. Bluestone established a hospital-based home care system at Montefiore Hospital in New York City. This prototype became known as the hospital without walls, from which no one would be excluded based on age or illness. These principles were later extended to the home setting, in which medical personnel began providing the same care procedures to people living at home. From this system came the permanent establishment of an array of modern home care services, including medical services, nursing, social services, transportation, and housekeeping (Spiegel, 1987).

Modern-Day Home Care

Home care has become a multifaceted industry, providing people with a variety of services and options necessary to maintain their ability to live at home. Today, home care encompasses more than just personal care (e.g., bathing, dressing, feeding). Rather, modern home care offers an array of services to care recipients and their families, including hospice services, the provision of necessary medical equipment (e.g., walkers, wheelchairs), respite care for family caregivers, companionship for care recipients, and mental health services (Buhler-Wilkerson, 2001).

Since the establishment of modern home care, several factors have influenced people to choose home care in the 21st century as an alternative to institutional care. Among these factors are economic and financial incentives that are making home care part of the mainstream of medical practice in the United States (Bishop, 2004). Care recipients and their families, along with physicians, hospital managers, and policymakers, have sought to improve and use home care options that may be more financially feasible for families and economically feasible for the health care system as a whole.

In addition to its cost-effectiveness, perhaps a predominant reason people choose to receive home care services in instances of illness, disability, or age-related complications is to help ensure and maintain a desired quality of life. Stein (2001) notes that home care strives to change both the locus and the focus of care, with the intention of removing care from an institutional setting and helping people maximize daily functioning and well-being in their homes. Many professional disciplines recognize the importance of emphasizing quality of life in conjunction with maintaining medical stability and have sought to expand their knowledge on how to ensure that a person's quality of life is sustained in the home care setting (Niewnhous, 2007).

Future Trends in Home Care

Although home health care has been common among past generations, it is becoming even more widespread in the United States as the American population continues to change in terms of numbers, diversity, and familial contexts (Buhler-Wilkerson, 2001; Veronesi, 2001). Expected among these trends is an increase in novel services such as long-distance caregiving. In many cases, family members and significant others live too far away to provide direct care themselves and therefore hire home care providers who are local to their loved one. Such services can range from personal care, to case management, to housekeeping services. Today, adult children and their parents are more likely than ever to live far apart for a variety of reasons, including job opportunities for the children and the parents' decision to relocate upon retirement. As a future trend in home care, long-distance caregiving is an emerging service gaining momentum (Smith, 2006).

As home care trends continue, continuity of care and adequate communication between various health professionals will demand greater attention. People receiving home care often receive a variety of other services, such as physical therapy, case management, and routine exams from a primary physician. For this reason, professionals from multidisciplinary services must continue to improve techniques that allow the proper exchange of information in order to optimize care in the home (Brown et al., 2006; Peters & McKeon, 1998).

STAFFING OF HOME CARE ORGANIZATIONS

Home care organizations vary in their size, structure, and services provided. Some agencies may consist of a single person providing a specific service (e.g., speech therapy), whereas other agencies may be much larger and offer a wide range of comprehensive services to home care recipients. It is important to understand the different types of organizations or agencies in the home care industry. In general, there are three categories of home care organizations or agencies (May, 1999; Montgomery, Holley, Deichert, & Kosloski, 2005): proprietary or for-profit, not-for-profit, and government or official agencies.

Proprietary or For-Profit Agencies

Agencies of this type are owned and operated by an individual or, in most cases, a business group or corporation. An individual or a board of directors serves as the governing body, and as the name implies, the goals of these agencies are to provide service to home care recipients and to make a profit for the individual owner or group. Most direct care workers (e.g., home health aides [HHAs]) work in for-profit agencies (61.5%), and a large number of workers (16.8%) are self-employed (May, 1999; Montgomery et al., 2005).

Not-for-Profit Agencies

Agencies of this type are privately owned, operated, and governed yet qualify for tax exemption because of their not-for-profit status. These agencies may be owned by individuals or groups, yet as their name implies they do not operate to generate profit. Voluntary agencies may also be included in the not-for-profit group. These groups differ in that they are governed by community-based groups, such as churches or charities. Approximately 10% of direct care workers are employed in the not-for-profit sector (May, 1999; Montgomery et al., 2005).

Government or Official Agencies

These agencies are administered by the state or local government and tend to focus on prevention and education as well as the provision of home care. Because these are government agencies, they are managed through departments of health or other government entities (e.g., county commissions). Approximately 11.4% of direct care workers are employed in government or official agencies (May, 1999; Montgomery et al., 2005).

Staffing in home care organizations tends to vary depending on the level of services offered. Some organizations provide a wide array of services through in-house employees or through a network of professions, whereas others provide limited services and may concentrate on one or two particular types of care, such as skilled nursing or the provision of medical equipment (e.g., hospital beds, oxygen tanks). Consequently, it is not surprising that some HHAs are trained as certified nursing assistants, able to provide some health care services, whereas other HHAs are less trained, do not provide medical services, and provide important help with instrumental activities such as shopping and cleaning. In general, the types of care available to those receiving services in the home are quite extensive and include medical care, nursing care, physical therapy, occupational therapy, respiratory therapy, speech therapy, psychosocial assessments and interventions, light house-keeping, cooking, shopping, medical equipment set-up and service, and friendly visiting.

Health Disciplines Represented in Home Care

Home care organizations generally are staffed or networked with people trained in a wide range of health disciplines, each responsible for a specific aspect of care (Hepburn & Keenan, 1997; May, 1999; National Association for Home Care and Hospice, 2007; Navarra & Ferrer, 1997). It is important to note that educating home care recipients and, in many cases, their family members is also an integral service that is provided by each of these disciplines because the overall goal of home care is to help people live as independently as possible. The health care disciplines represented in home care are as follows.

Medicine

Although physicians and nurse practitioners differ in their professional training and licensing, this group is generally responsible for assessing the physical well-being of care recipients, making medical diagnoses, prescribing medical interventions, and setting courses of treatment within the overall plan of care. Typically, they provide medical services through a network or through referral rather than through a home care agency itself. Home care recipients typically do not obtain physician services directly through home care agencies (only 2.4% do so); rather, they continue to see their own physicians, who supervise their care and coordinate services with the home care agencies (Table 4.1). Physicians also may serve as medical directors of larger, more diversified home care organizations. In this role, the physician's responsibilities extend beyond typical duties and include planning and management activities along with the leadership of the medical team.

Nursing

The various types of nurses are distinguished by their levels of training and licensing, and their job duties differ greatly. Registered nurses (RNs) are responsible for assessing patients, making nursing and treatment diagnoses (nonmedical), moni-

toring physical conditions, administering medications, and providing skilled nursing services, such as intravenous care. RNs also typically serve as the primary liaison between the physician and the home care recipient. RNs dictate and supervise
the nursing care provided by other levels of nursing. Licensed practical nurses
(LPNs) or licensed vocational nurses (LVNs) are people who have received
less technical education than RNs but have passed state licensing requirements.
LPNs are responsible for routine skilled nursing care (e.g., wound care, medication
administration) and may supervise the care provided by HHAs. HHAs are people
who have completed a minimal level of nursing training and have obtained certification to provide nursing care. HHAs provide a wide range of services, including
assistance with bathing, dressing, meals, and ambulating, changing bed linens and
cleaning portable commodes, assisting with transfers from bed to wheelchair, and
performing exercises as prescribed by therapists. HHAs may also provide light
housekeeping services. The majority of home care recipients (75.0%) need skilled
nursing services such as wound care or the administration of medicine (Table 4.1).
A significant percentage of home care recipients also need assistance with per-

Table 4.1. Service Use by Home Care Clients ($N = 1,355,300$)

Services	% of Clients Who Use Service
Medical and skilled nursing	
Physician	2.4
Skilled nursing	75.0
Equipment and medication	
Medical equipment	8.1
Medications	6.6
Personal care	
Continuous home care	3.9
Companionship	3.0
Housekeeping	24.3
Personal care	35.1
Transportation	1.9
Respite care	1.3
Therapeutic	
Dietary or nutritional	4.4
Intravenous therapy	3.9
Occupational therapy	8.3
Physical therapy	26.6
Respiratory therapy	2.2
Speech and audiology therapy	2.3
Psychosocial	
Counseling	1.7
Psychological	1.1
Social	8.7
Spiritual or pastoral	1.1
Referral	2.6

Source: Centers for Disease Control (2004).
Note: Data derived from the 2000 U.S. Census.

sonal care (35.1%) and housekeeping (24.3%). Typically, clients need some combination of skilled nursing services and personal care, along with other therapies (e.g., physical therapy). Because nursing constitutes the majority of the services provided through home care organizations, agency staffs consist largely of RNs, LPNs, LVNs, and HHAs.

Rehabilitation Therapy

A wide array of rehabilitation therapies are offered through home care organizations because the therapeutic needs of home care recipients are diverse. Each specialist is educated and licensed to perform her or his particular area of therapy. Therapists may be employed by the home care agency or, more commonly, contracted out through a network of providers. Physical therapists (PTs) conduct assessments and evaluate the physical needs and goals of clients, develop interventions, and provide therapy. PTs commonly work with home care recipients to increase strength, balance, and coordination after hospitalizations and surgeries (e.g., hip replacements); 26.6% of home care patients need physical therapy (Table 4.1).

Occupational therapists (OTs) are concerned with the functional status of home care recipients in terms of their ability to perform ADLs such as toileting, eating, dressing, bathing, and transferring (e.g., bed to wheelchair, wheelchair to commode). Approximately 8.3% of home care recipients need the services of OTs. Respiratory therapists (RTs) administer respiratory tests, care, and treatments, such as the use of ventilators, oxygen equipment, and other breathing supplies. Approximately 2.2% of home care recipients need respiratory therapy. Speech therapists (speech–language pathologists) assist home care recipients with speech and language deficits, difficulties with swallowing or positioning, and cognitive deficits that may affect communication or eating. Approximately 2.3% of home care recipients use the services of speech–language pathologists.

Social Work

Social workers in the context of home care are responsible primarily for the logistical aspects of caregiving, such as locating and arranging for necessary services and resources, assisting clients with insurance paperwork, and applying for government assistance. Social workers may also provide assessment, counseling, crisis intervention, advocacy, and mediation services to clients and their families. Approximately 8.7% of home care recipients use social services, with an additional 1.7% needing some form of counseling. Counseling and psychological services may also be provided by psychologists or psychiatric nurses.

Ancillary Services

A variety of secondary or ancillary services are also available through home care organizations. These include the services of dietitians and nutritionists, pharmacists, medical equipment technicians, housekeepers, companions or sitters, and volunteers. Home care recipients commonly use ancillary services, typically in combination with other services.

Because the staffing of home care organizations reflects the needs of the clients, it is important to understand the characteristics of current home care clients and the projected characteristics of clients of the near future. Skilled nursing care is the predominant need of home care recipients (Table 4.1), yet a great deal of diversity exists in terms of services needed. As the baby boom generation enters later life and as the U.S. population lives longer and with higher levels of chronic illness, the needs of home care clients probably will increase in volume and intensity. The desire of clients to be treated at home and the cost-effectiveness of home care will drive the staffing of organizations and may lead to an expansion of services to include all but the most technical aspects of medical care.

EMPOWERING HOME CARE
WORKERS, CLIENTS, AND FAMILIES

This section provides a discussion of the empowerment of HHAs, followed by a consideration of EWTs as a means of empowering HHAs and finally the empowerment of home care recipients and family members. Despite the variety of home care organizations, most agencies tend to be structured in the traditional pyramid shape. The hierarchy of the health care field has largely dictated the structure of home care organizations, with physicians in the decision-making role at the top of the pyramid, RNs and therapists at the managerial level, and LPNs and HHAs at the base of the pyramid. Physicians diagnose and prescribe care, RNs and therapists draft care plans, and LPNs and HHAs execute the care plans. As is typical of the pyramid structure, information and ideas flow downward, and rarely do LPNs or HHAs have input into the decision-making process or the manner in which work is performed. Certainly, the typical structure of home care organizations appears to be contrary to the goal of client-centered service in that those who may know the client best (e.g., LPNs, HHAs) typically cannot relay information about the client to those with the capacity to make decisions and changes in the plan of care.

This limitation raises the question of precisely how to create an empowered workplace in home care, particularly given the entrenched hierarchal structure. The first step in empowering workers is to create an environment that facilitates communication and the exchange of information. This includes not only the information HHAs have about clients and the work HHAs perform but also information they do not have about management operations, such as the costs of doing business. A transparent approach to information sharing allows all levels of the organization to better understand how and why certain decisions are made and encourages creative and novel approaches (Sagie & Koslowsky, 2000).

In home care organizations, several steps can be taken to open lines of communication and increase employee participation in decision-making processes. Care plans drive the services that home care clients receive and largely dictate the work performed by home care workers. Home care organizations can enhance direct care workers' sense of empowerment by soliciting their input in the development of care plans and listening to HHAs as they report back on the status of clients. Ideally, care plans change as the needs of clients change, and direct care workers often are situated to assist in the adjustment of care plans because of their high level of client contact. Including HHAs in interdisciplinary team meetings can also enhance communication and provide a venue for workers to express opinions and ideas that may lead to improved service. Home care organizations may also choose to include direct care workers on committees that formulate policy and control future directions for the agency. Finally, providing HHAs with information about actions taken by the organization can increase their sense of control and alleviate fears of the unknown (e.g., the financial stability of the organization, the discontinuation of certain services). Improving communication and sharing information are essential steps in the empowerment process and a suitable starting point for home care organizations looking to expand and improve the roles of direct care workers.

Sharing and delegating responsibilities for decision making are two additional actions that can empower workers. Both sharing and delegating responsibility involve the transfer of power from management to the HHAs. In sharing responsibility, management relinquishes a degree of decision-making authority to the workers, resulting in joint decision making. In delegation, management completely relinquishes decision-making authority to the HHAs. Successful transfer of power depends heavily on strong communication, information sharing, a competent workforce, and a commitment of trust between management and HHAs. Transfer of decision-making authority can benefit both the organization and the workers. Management may be freed from the burden of making lower-level decisions, allowing them to focus on higher-level duties such as business development. HHAs may be empowered as they gain feelings of enhanced autonomy and locus of control (Sagie & Koslowsky, 2000).

A number of opportunities exist in home care organizations to share and delegate decision making. The first step in this process is to consider precisely what types of decisions can be shared with or made by direct care workers. Certain decisions, such as medication management, are dictated by legal standards and are not subject to sharing or delegation. However, many other decisions can and should be delegated to some extent to direct care workers. For example, the timing of care (e.g., bathing times, meal times) or the degree to which direct care workers incorporate the assistance of spouses or family members into the caregiving regimen are decisions that are best made by the workers or in consultation with management. Management can also build options into care plans that allow HHAs to make decisions as they see fit, depending on the conditions they encounter in the field. For instance, providing HHAs with a choice of range-of-motion exercises allows them to tailor the intervention depending on the status or desires of the client on any given day. Again, delegating authority to any degree relies on the competence of the workers and the confidence that management has in the workers to make appropriate decisions. It also relies heavily on the notion that the HHA is the person most familiar with clients' situations and that HHAs are best qualified to make certain decisions. Again, the sharing and delegation of decision-making power to direct care workers can have several significant bene-fits, including the creation of a cooperative workplace, better time management, and, ultimately, better home care service.

Finally, HHAs can be empowered when they are provided with opportunities for advancement and the ability to share in the rewards of success. For HHAs in home care, this means providing them with time, resources, and encouragement to gain additional training necessary for professional advancement. Home care or-ganizations can allot time for workers to attend formal training courses for contin-uing education credits or provide tuition reimbursement for workers attending technical schools or universities. In doing so, home care organizations are not only empowering workers with knowledge and opportunity (see Chapter 8) but also reaping the rewards of a better-trained workforce.

Home care organizations can also allow HHAs to share in the success of the organization through profit-sharing or performance-based compensation. These actions provide workers with a direct, concrete link between the quality of their work and the rewards they receive. When workers are empowered with a sense of ownership, they may feel more compelled to use better and more creative problem-solving methods and to seek out more cost-effective means of achieving success (Potterfield, 1999). In addition to the obvious benefits that this form of empower-ment provides to the HHAs and to the home care organization, better service to the home care recipient is an important byproduct of this process.

At first glance, the benefits of empowering HHAs in home care organizations appear to be obvious and simple to achieve. However, several factors can impede such efforts. As mentioned earlier, the health care profession is marked by a fairly regimented hierarchal structure. It may be a challenge for home care organizations to break down this hierarchy and to change existing power dynamics. Second, home care organizations tend to be decentralized in terms of home offices and places of practice. Because care is delivered in the home setting rather than in a central location (e.g., hospital, nursing home), it can be difficult to promote effec-tive communication between health care professionals or facilitate a team ap-proach to decision making. Finally, empowering home care workers may entail a change in the way in which organizations view HHAs. Turnover is high among HHAs, and organizations may view them as replaceable and unworthy of invest-ments in trust, training, or additional compensation. Trusting and valuing work-ers is essential and may indeed be the first step for home care organizations to take on their way to creating an empowered workplace.

Potential of EWTs in Home Care

The preceding discussions of the historical and structural context of home care and empowerment in home care suggest that the home care milieu is fertile ground for the potential benefits of EWTs. However, the use of EWTs in home care organi-zations has not been formally attempted to our knowledge, nor has there been a formal evaluation of EWTs in the home care setting.

EWTs in the home care setting probably would be limited to home care organizations that are large enough to support a group of HHAs responsible for serving people in their homes. In smaller organizations that do not support enough HHAs to create a team, it appears that simply empowering the individuals themselves would provide many of the same benefits found in EWTs. In a home care organization that can support an EWT, the team would have many of the same benefits as those found for direct care workers in nursing homes and perhaps others as well. The EWT would allow the HHAs to meet regularly and share problems, frustrations, and solutions. Currently, HHAs work very independently and typically do not have regular opportunities to share experiences and learn from one another. This includes teaching one another what works and what does not work when providing service in the home care environment.

The EWTs would also facilitate communication and information exchange between the HHAs and others in the home care organization. Because the HHAs work in individual homes, communication with one another and with other staff of the home care organization is not always easy to accomplish. The EWT would facilitate regular interaction between the managers of the home care organization and the HHAs. This would allow managers to get input from the EWT on management decisions to be made or to turn over some decision making to the team. With regard to participating in decision making, examples include allowing the HHAs to determine who will serve which home care residents, to determine who will receive days off for holidays, and to provide input about health care plans.

Implementing EWTs among HHAs probably would follow procedures similar to those for other direct care workers (see Part III and the Appendix for details). This would include initial planning and orientation of the staff so that everyone understands the value of the EWTs and responsibilities related to them. It would also include training for management, the HHAs, a team facilitator, and other staff so that they are able to carry out their new roles. The HHAs would learn how to interact in team meetings, follow an agenda, and take notes. The managers would learn ways of involving the HHAs in decision making and the importance of obtaining regular input from the HHAs and providing meaningful feedback.

Empowering Clients and Families

In the home health care environment, the advantages of empowerment apply not only to HHAs but also to other stakeholders in the home health care industry. This includes the people receiving the care and informal (i.e., unpaid) caregivers, such as family members and significant others (Magaziner et al., 2000). Such an expanded empowerment model would allow an increasingly client-centered approach to home care.

One substantial means of empowering residents and family members that has been implemented is the Cash and Counseling Demonstration and Evaluation (CCDE; Gaugler & Teaster, 2006, pp. 145–146). The CCDE empowers residents in that it offers older adults the ability to hire family members to provide needed home health care services. Early demonstration efforts provided Medicaid consumers with cash and counseling services in Florida, Arkansas, and New Jersey; cash allowances were provided along with information (Simon-Rusinowitz, Mahoney, Loughlin, & DeBarthe Sadler, 2005). Older consumers retained flexibility in the services they could purchase, which ranged from home care to other options, such as home modification. In an example of how CCDE could be considered an "empowerment" community-based long-term care model, training was provided to consumers in the hiring, retention, payment, and management of care providers.

Existing data on the evaluation of CCDE in Arkansas found that this model had a range of benefits for home care recipients and their family caregivers, including relief of work and financial strain for family caregivers, the opportunity to supplement existing informal care, high satisfaction, reduction in unmet care needs, and a modest reduction in nursing home admissions (Dale & Brown, 2006; Dale, Brown, Phillips, Schore, & Carlson, 2003; Foster, Brown, Phillips, & Carlson, 2005; Simon-Rusinowitz et al., 2005). These findings suggest that in home care settings, it can be beneficial to expand empowerment beyond the HHAs to include the clients.

In sum, the preliminary findings of EWTs in nursing homes and the CCDE suggest that improved care can be achieved through empowered direct care workers, clients, and family members. Once the concept of empowerment is understood in home care, intervention approaches to improve empowerment such as EWTs among HHAs and CCDE for residents can be implemented. With this new focus on empowerment, outcomes such as improved resident care can be expected. And it is not unreasonable to suspect that these could lead to desirable delays in nursing home admission as well (Brod, Stewart, Sands, & Walton, 1999; Gaugler, Kane, & Langlois, 2000; Logsdon, Gibbons, McCurry, & Teri, 1999).

As research and our understanding of long-term care have advanced, a rising chorus of voices have called for the empowerment of direct care workers and residents as a means of achieving client-centered care and moving away from the institutionalized, medicalized model of care. Clearly, empowered direct care staff, who are in the closest day-to-day contact with older people, can positively affect health care decisions, which in turn can result in more appropriate and efficacious care delivery. However, there is still much room for in-depth studies of the empowerment process and the implementation of EWTs in the home care setting. With such study, EWTs and empowered residents can have a positive impact on home care staff, on the people receiving home care, and on the caregiving families and significant others.

PART II

Research Findings on the Effects of Empowered Work Teams and Empowerment in Long-Term Care

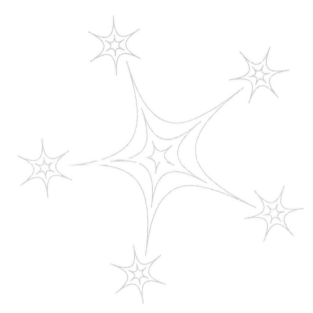

Although there have been numerous studies examining the effects of empowered work teams (EWTs) and empowerment in manufacturing settings, few have been conducted in health care and fewer still in long-term care. Chapter 5 provides a qualitative description of the implementation and effects of EWTs in the Green House project, inspired by Robert Thomas. Chapter 6 reviews a longitudinal study examining the impacts of EWTs on resident care, job attitudes, and turnover in four nursing homes compared with four conventional nursing homes without EWTs. Chapter 7 examines the effects of EWTs on direct care worker turnover and on work performance and job attitudes. Chapter 8 examines the impacts of education and training on employee empowerment.

CHAPTER 5

The Effects of Empowered Work Teams in the Green House Project

Jude Rabig

Being a Shahbaz has empowered me and the people I work with. It has boosted our self esteem, our work confidence, and it has given us pride to come to work every day to give the proper care to the people we work with. We have been empowered through this opportunity. They have taken us, the bottom of the employment chain, and allowed us to move up to the front. . . . We have harmony and it works. If I said the transition was easy I wouldn't be being honest, because it was a whole change of life. But we learned from our mistakes and from those who had more experience than us.

—Bridget Bumphis, Shahbaz
Green House Project Symposium
March 21, 2005, Tupelo, MS

The implementation of empowered work teams (EWTs) in the Green House Project was a complex and challenging venture. It challenged project leaders to develop a structure and training that had not been envisioned before. It represented for the staff a dramatic shift in their philosophy and work practices and a substantial change in the individuals' roles and responsibilities within the organization.

The Green House Project was based on a conceptual model developed by culture change leader William Thomas. It represented his emergent thinking about the failure of the traditional medical-model skilled nursing home to provide quality of life or quality of care for older adults. For almost a decade his Eden Alternative movement had attempted to improve nursing home quality of life, but the work was challenging and the system resistant to change. Green House was to be a radical redesign that reconfigured the architecture, changed the core philosophy, and reorganized the staffing model of the traditional skilled nursing home. The operating unit is one house of 10 older adults with a rich staffing pattern of well-educated direct care workers. Several houses represented one licensed nursing home. The habilitative philosophy recognized the resident not as a passive, sick person but as an active participant in the household (Rabig, Thomas, Kane, Cutler, & McAlilly, 2006).

The challenge was to transform Thomas's vision into practice within the regulatory and financial framework of skilled nursing. Funding to implement the project at a pilot site was provided by a grant from the Robert Wood Johnson

Foundation. The Green House pilot project site was the Cedars, a 120-bed skilled nursing home in Tupelo, Mississippi. Part of the Traceway Retirement Community, one of the four campuses in the Mississippi Methodist Senior Services system, the Cedars nursing home was old and slated for replacement. Jude Rabig, National Green House Project executive director, and Steve McAlilly, CEO of Mississippi Methodist Senior Services, were responsible for project implementation. The plan was to replace Cedars in two phases.

IN THE BEGINNING

In Phase 1, four houses were built. Each house had a living room, dining room, kitchen (collectively called the hearth), utility area, spa, office, den, fenced patio area, and 10 private resident rooms with baths. The houses met state and federal construction and operating regulations. The model also included electronic medical records, a pager call system, a two-way radio and beeper system, an alarmed egress front door, and in-house meal planning and preparation. One goal of the model was to create a work life for direct care staff that provided safety, empowerment, satisfaction, and competence. The environmental design consciously incorporated worker safety features. Ceiling lifts were provided to eliminate heavy lifting, bathrooms were configured to facilitate safe, easy showering, convenient storage and small-scale design minimized walking distances, and carts were eliminated.

The staffing reorganization created universal workers. Thomas coined the title *Shahbaz* to describe a direct care worker who was a certified nursing assistant (CNA) with 120 hours of additional training (Exhibit 5A). These workers would run the household in the most meaningful ways by doing the cooking, light cleaning, laundry, and elder care. Extensive research was done to identify the organizational structure the houses would use. The EWT was selected (Yeatts & Hyten, 1998). *Shahbaz* is a Persian word that means "royal falcon" and is intended to convey the importance of the role of the individuals who watch over the elders.

The project engaged Dale Yeatts as a consultant. He shared his expertise and provided technical assistance as the EWTs were being integrated into the Green House model. He also provided on-site consultation and training for project leaders and direct care staff. The Green House was to have an EWT of Shahbazim. They would be coached by a licensed nursing home administrator (LNHA), called the Guide, who would retain responsibility for ensuring that all nursing home regulations were met. Nurses and other clinical personnel were to form their own empowered teams, which worked collaboratively with the team of Shahbazim (Figure 5.1).

The initial task of the implementation was to identify those among the Cedars' existing staff who were interested in working in Green Houses. The first step was to educate all staff in the facility about the Green House model. This was achieved in 1-hour sessions that presented the vision and provided opportunity for discussion and questions. A job description of the new position was provided (Exhibit 5B), and a description of the training that a Shahbaz would need to complete was distributed. All staff members were invited to become Shahbazim. Thirty-six

EXHIBIT 5A.
Team Training Modules

1. Communications Skills (8 hrs)
   - Positive communication techniques
   - Communicating with residents
   - Understanding families

2. Autonomy and Choice (8 hrs)
   - Discuss autonomy
   - Restoring choice with attention to safety
   - Depression and its role in choice and decision making
   - Dementia and choice

3. Self-Managed Work Teams (16 hrs)
   - Meaning of self-managed work teams
   - Roll of the Guide (licensed nursing home administrator)
   - Characteristics of successful teams
   - Consensus
   - Collaboration
   - The team meeting
   - The code of ethics
   - Self-scheduling
   - Self-monitoring: use of team coordinators and checklists

4. Green House Operations (20 hrs)
   - Special policies and procedures
   - Activities in the greenhouse
   - Emergency management
   - Habilitation and adaptive devices
   - Visitors and families
   - Elders in the kitchen
   - Ceremony and celebration
   - Care planning
   - Pain management
   - Alternative therapies

(continued)

EXHIBIT 5A. *(continued)*

5. House Orientation and Training (4 hrs)

- House systems orientation
- Lift operation technology
- Pagers, alarms, and call systems
- Phones
- Appliances
- Supply ordering systems
- Housekeeping scheduling and techniques: policies reviewed

6. Culinary Training (40 hrs)

- Serve-safe training
- Menu planning
- Software for ordering food
- Nutrition and dietary adjustments
- Measuring
- Basic preparation techniques
- Serving
- Clean up

7. Emergency Management (24 hrs)

- CPR
- First aid
- Emergency protocols

---

positions were available, and 20 people indicated a desire to be trained: 18 certified nursing assistants, 1 cook, and 1 housekeeper. Any staff member who indicated a desire to train for the new position was placed on the staff list. The plan was to grant positions to staff based on seniority. No supervisor input was sought, nor were internal candidates screened. This was based on the philosophy that individuals possess the best understanding of their own capacity and that interest and motivation are key factors in success.

Because not all available positions were filled through this internal recruitment process, outside candidates were sought through newspaper advertisements. Twelve external candidates were selected; none had prior health care experience. CNA training was provided for any worker who was not already a CNA.

Four EWTs were formed in the pilot project, one for each Green House. Teams consisted of five core staff and sufficient part-time and relief staff. The

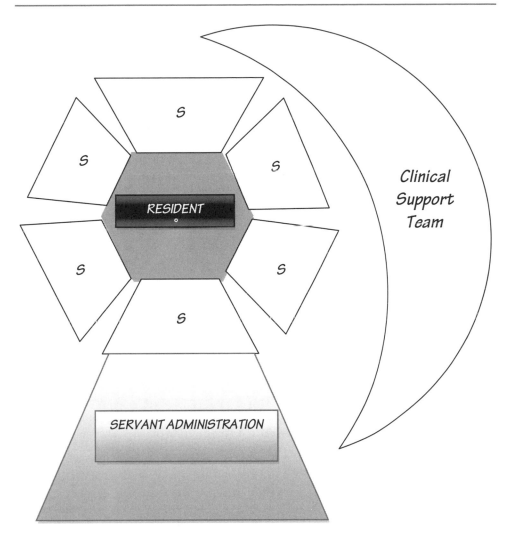

Figure 5.1. Organizational Design of a Team of Shahbazim. *Note:* S = Shahbaz.

staffing pattern in each house is two Shahbazim on the day and evening shifts and one on the night shift. The average team size was eight or nine Shahbazim. Every effort was made to honor staff requests for assignment to a particular team. The most common requests focused not on a desire to work with particular peers but rather on a desire to continue to take care of familiar residents. This request was made most frequently by the staff from the special care dementia unit. These requests were honored through adjustment of the matrix of residents and staff assigned to individual houses.

Training curricula were created for the education of all staff who would be participating in the Green Houses. The staff modules were based on an understanding of the participants' current level of knowledge compared with what they would need to know to work effectively in the new model and on an assessment of the existing organizational dynamics. On-site observations, small focus groups, and individual meetings were held to complete this assessment. This revealed the

EXHIBIT 5B.
Job Description (Shahbaz)

QUALIFICATIONS

An applicant should have an interest in caring for elders, a willingness to work as a member of a team, and an understanding of the requirements of the position.

A.   Education

A Shahbaz will complete

1.   CNA course

2.   Serve safe course, or other state-approved food-handling course

3.   CPR certification

4.   First aid course from American Red Cross or American Heart Association

5.   Green House Shahbaz Training Program (40 hours)

6.   Culinary training

An individual may work in a Green House under the direction of a fully trained Shahbaz after completing 1 and 5, but may not engage food preparation or emergency management.

B.   Skills Required

The following are skills needed to perform, with or without reasonable accommodation, the essential functions of providing care to elders. The ability to

- Recognize the autonomy and dignity of all elders.

- Communicate a sense of caring, concern and dignity for elders.

- Understand how to place decision making in the hands of the elders whenever possible and appropriate.

- Make prompt and accurate judgments with regard to elder care and emergencies.

- Work and communicate effectively as part of the self managed work team.

C.   Duties and Responsibilities

The Shahbaz will provide care to the elders living in a Green House. Their primary role is to protect, sustain, and nurture the elders by providing assistance with activities of daily living and meeting other needs as required. The core goal of the work of the Shahbaz will be to provide assistance that promotes a high quality of life and a positive elderhood. The responsibilities of the Shahbaz include care of the elder and the elder's environment, in-

EXHIBIT 5B. *(continued)*

cluding cooking, laundry, and housekeeping. The Shahbaz is a member of a self-managed work team and is responsible for coordinating aspects of the team's work.

D.   Functions of the Job

- Recognize and respond to the needs of elders.

- Promote autonomy of elders in decision making.

- Report changes in the elder's condition to the clinical support team per Green House change in condition protocols.

- Assist elder with personal care functions, including

  – Dental and mouth care

  – Bathing

  – Dressing and grooming

  – Hair care

  – Nail care

  – Shaving

  – Bowel and bladder care

  – Other personal and hygiene care

- Observe and report the presence of pressure areas to prevent decubitus and provide skin care according to policy.

- Make occupied and unoccupied beds and change bed linens.

- Assist moving, positioning, and transporting elders into and out of beds, chairs, bathtubs, wheelchairs, lifts, etc.

- Ensure that call bracelet is being worn by the elder at all times and answered promptly.

- Communicate with co-workers at all levels to adequately meet the needs of elders.

- Meet with the clinical support team as scheduled or needed to discuss elders' needs and progress in identifying and correcting problems.

- Report accidents and incidents when they occur.

- Maintain a lift-free environment.

- Assist with or perform restorative and rehabilitative procedures as outlined by the care plan.

- Measure and record vital signs, such as temperature, pulse, respirations, weight, height, anatomical dimension, and circumference.

- Report any resident abuse or suspected abuse to the Guide immediately.

(continued)

EXHIBIT 5B. (*continued*)

- Assist with the application of slings, elastic bandages, binders, etc.

- Provide range-of-motion exercises.

- Observe, monitor, and report to the clinical support team any change in condition, using the Green House change in condition protocols.

- Attend and participate in orientation programs, ongoing training, and educational classes.

- Follow established safety precautions and observe, monitor, and intervene or report to the Guide unsafe conditions in the Green House.

- Follow established smoking regulations and report violations.

- Maintain confidentiality and privacy of elder care, procedures, and documentation.

- Prepare, serve, and clean up after meals and snacks.

- Launder clothing, linen, and other articles.

- Clean and maintain the environment of the Green House.

- Observe standard precautions per Green House policy.

- Document observed data per organization policy.

- Keep all areas of the Green House clean.

- Prepare and serve meals, between meal, bedtime, and other nutritional snacks per the posted menu and the stated preferences of the elder.

- Perform routine housekeeping duties.

- Perform other related duties as needed by the elder.

ACCOUNTABILITY

The Shahbaz works cooperatively with other Shahbazim on the Green House self-managed work team. The team and individual Shahbaz work collaboratively with the clinical support team (CST). The CST directs all matters related to skilled nursing services. The self-managed work team and individual Shahbaz report to the Green House Guide in all other matters. The Shahbazim seek counsel and assistance with problem solving from the Sage.

---

pre–Green House structure to have a fairly typical nursing home organizational dynamic. There was a steep bureaucracy and poor communication. Information flow usually was top down and one way; it focused on direction and supervision, with very little communication and information sharing. Information was owned by management. Memos and directives that cluttered the bulletin boards were the only secondary form of communication used in the organization. High levels of distrust were endemic and most intense in the nurse–direct care worker relationship. The direct care workers reported feeling that they were not respected by their supervisors, that their work was not valued, and that they were perceived as dispensable and easy to replace. These findings and the functional model of the EWT helped to form the training objectives.

Improvements were needed to foster the development of teams. Training modules were developed that would allow all learners to

- know the differences between collaboration and other types of work relationships;

- identify the potential benefits of collaboration in the Green House;

- know the differences between majority rule and consensus;

- demonstrate the ability to participate successfully in the group process to reach consensus;

- use brainstorming and critical thinking to solve problems;

- communicate effectively with peers and leaders.

The team was intended to have more responsibility than an empowered direct care worker team in a traditional nursing home. The vast array of tasks to be completed in each house made it difficult to envision one individual Shahbaz accepting the role of team leader. Analyses of the work led us to create five coordinator roles on each team. A housekeeping coordinator, food coordinator, team coordinator, care coordinator, and scheduling coordinator were established. Team members selected the people from the team to fill these roles.

The *housekeeping coordinator* was responsible for monitoring the overall cleanliness of the house and ordering cleaning supplies.

The *food coordinator* organized the menu planning meeting with residents and staff, reviewed the menus with the dietitian, ordered food, reviewed food intake, and tracked residents' weights.

The *scheduling coordinator* gathered team schedule requests at the team meeting and created a draft schedule for discussion and approval by the team at the next meeting. Once a schedule was approved by the team, if a team member could not be at work it was the team member's responsibility to find a replacement. In emergencies, the scheduling coordinator would find a replacement.

The *care coordinator* was responsible for monitoring the team's compliance with the care plan. They checked that the care was given and documented. They collaborated with the clinical support team (CST) when CST members (e.g., nurses, physicians, medical specialists) visited the houses.

The *team coordinator* was responsible for planning the team meetings, posting the agenda, leading the meeting, and communicating team decisions to the team Guide, CST, and families.

The coordinators served for at least 1 month but not more than 3 months. Each member was expected to eventually rotate through each coordinator position.

This was intended to teach all team members the full range of roles and responsibilities and to create empathy among the coordinators. This division of responsibility worked well. After implementation, Shahbazim said that they were patient with their peers because, as one Shahbaz reported, "I knew I would be doing the coordinating in a few months, and I wanted everyone to cooperate with me when I was responsible." This arrangement also gave each team member a deeper understanding of all operational issues in the house.

The team meeting was designed to be the formal mechanism for running the household. Decisions were to be made, problems solved, and controversies resolved during the team meeting. It was scheduled as a weekly event, usually for 1 hour, to be held at a time, date, and location to be determined by the team. CST members monitored the house so that Shahbazim could meet. An agenda for the meeting was posted in the office, and those who wanted to bring something to the team for discussion or problem solving could place it on the agenda as long as they signed their name. Before the meeting, the team coordinator met with the Guide, prioritized the agenda items, and allocated a specific amount of time for discussion. The team coordinator also clarified any unclear agenda items with the person who posted them. Only the Guide and the team attended the meetings unless other staff were invited by the team. All meetings began with a reading of the code of ethics (Exhibit 5C). Standard agenda items included a monthly house budget report, a monthly discussion of learning needs to plan staff development, achievements to celebrate, and improvements to consider. Additional items were added to the agenda by anyone who wanted to add a topic, including residents, families, and other staff. The meeting process was fairly formal. Each agenda item was read, and all members in turn spoke on the item or issue. No one was allowed to interrupt a team member who was speaking, and no one could comment in between speakers. Ideas or potential solutions were recorded as presented. Each idea was then individually put to the group for a consensus vote. Members used the "rule of thumb" hand signals: thumbs up for "yes," thumbs down for "no," and thumbs sideways for "I can live with it" (Yeatts & Hyten, 1998). Any idea that got even a single "thumbs down" was eliminated as a possible solution. If several ideas achieved consensus, to arrive at the final solution, a traditional vote was taken to determine which of the solutions was most popular. Any resolution of agenda items that pertained to others not present at the meeting was communicated to non–team members by the team coordinator after the meeting, and the agenda and minutes were placed in a house communication notebook for those who missed the meeting.

A team charter was developed that included the mission and values, key customers, guiding principles, and time commitments of the team (Fisher, Rayner, & Belgard, 1995). The mission of the team was defined by leaders as follows: "The Self Managed work team will protect, sustain and nurture the elders of the Green House by providing support and assistance with activities of daily living including personal care and nursing care as outlined by the clinical support team."

The team charter provided policies, procedures, and parameters for the teams' work and schedules. During their training, each team learned and practiced the process for team meetings, including reaching consensus. And each team was given a thorough understanding of the team's mission.

In an effort to enhance ownership of the team model, the teams were asked to create their own codes of ethics. They were given information about the purpose of a code of ethics, and they reviewed several codes from other professions such as accountants and firefighters. They were asked to hold team meetings to write their codes, and they were asked to reach consensus. This process took more than 4 hours. The teams were serious and thoughtful, and they worked diligently. At the end of the work the four teams were brought together to share their codes. The similarities were striking. The codes were discussed, and it was determined by consensus that the houses should share a single code of ethics. The codes were blended, and consensus was reached on inclusion of items and language (Exhibit 5C). The code subsequently served as a key component of the team charter.

Because of the newness of the Green House operation and the heavy regulatory burden under which nursing homes operate, the mechanism for monitoring work performance was not left for the team to create. Rather, it was provided to the team. A set of checklists was created for each team coordinator to complete at prescribed times, usually daily. These checklists provided the means for evaluating

---

EXHIBIT 5C.
Shahbazim Code of Ethics

A Shahbaz will work with others as a respectful, supportive, and flexible team member.

A Shahbaz will keep his or her word.

A Shahbaz is dependable, honest, and trustworthy.

A Shahbaz continues to grow, learn, and be committed to the well-being of elders.

A Shahbaz includes elders in decision making as much as possible.

A Shahbaz never crosses the line between providing care and providing clinical treatment.

A Shahbaz is patient with elders, with others, and with all members of the organization and community who come to the Green House.

A Shahbaz is a good communicator.

A Shahbaz shows responsibility to the elders and to the other members of the team by practicing good work habits, including

- coming in when scheduled and being on time;

- completing his or her work;

- leaving personal problems at home;

- giving complete reports about the elders to the other Shahbazim.

---

the teams' performance. Furthermore, the team Guide met every 1 or 2 days with the coordinators to discuss the house's performance.

STAGES OF EMPOWERED WORK TEAM DEVELOPMENT

Various authors (Schroder, 1963; Smith, 1960; Tuckman, 1965) have suggested phases of team development. Observations of the teams in Tupelo paralleled the Tuckman (1965) model of forming, storming, norming, and performing. The groups moved through these stages not in a linear consistent way but rather in an inconsistent manner that exhibited characteristics of one stage, then another, then a return to the first, with an overall trending from phase to phase. Teams began to work together 6 weeks before the move to the Green Houses. They prepared residents for the moves, met with families, and prepared the houses.

For the first 1–2 months groups were quiet and performed in a way that met objectives but did not exceed them. They were transitioning from working as individuals to working as part of a team, and they were deciding how to accomplish tasks. Questions such as who would cook and who would do housework became major issues of discussion. Often they led to tension and anxiety, and not infrequently team members asked the Guide to make decisions that belonged to the team. There was a need for the Guide to consistently direct the decision making back to the team members and to coach them while they solved the problems. There was hesitant and cautious participation at meetings, and members needed frequent coaching and support from the Guide on the processes associated with teamwork.

By the third month one of the four teams was fully engaged in substantial intragroup conflict. There was defensiveness, competition, and jealousy between members, anxiety, and a great deal of arguing. By the fourth month all four teams were in a similar state. Some team members were hostile or overzealous in expressing their individuality and resisting group formation. One team member resigned her position during this phase, stating that she preferred working on her own, and another member switched houses because she could not meld with her original team. This was a positive change, and she adapted to the new team quite quickly. There were sharp fluctuations in individual feelings and interpersonal relationships from day to day. There were petty arguments and disunity. Each team needed the Guide's attention each day. This stage called for the Guide to exhibit patience and to have coaching and mentoring skills. One Guide, who eventually left the project, continually fell back into an authoritarian management style. He made decisions for the team, reprimanded members for actions, and set goals without team input. This escalated the team's storming behaviors. Eventually, with a new Guide in place the teams began to develop trust, fine tune communication skills, and learn how to hold each member of the team accountable for the team outcomes. The storming period lasted for varying lengths of time. One team began the quiet stage of performing after 2 months of storming; another took fully 8 months to reach the performing stage.

By the end of the first year all four teams were able to communicate well, hold productive team meetings, and solve problems, often without assistance, and they exhibited improved levels of critical thinking skills.

It is important to note that while the teams' dynamics were emerging and they were progressing through their development, the work in the houses was being accomplished in an acceptable manner. Evaluations by the Guide, residents, and families indicated a high level of confidence and satisfaction in the teams' performance as it related to the residents and the household, even when high levels of interpersonal conflict were present.

EVALUATION AND IMPROVEMENT
OF THE IMPLEMENTATION PROCESS

Because this was a pilot project, ongoing evaluations of the teams and their effectiveness were conducted. The evaluation was meant to be formative, that is, it sought to learn how the program and its implementation could improve. Regular observations and meetings with the participants and residents contributed to the understanding of the project. The teams were considered one of the strongest, most important components of the Green Houses. Shahbazim reported high levels of satisfaction and empowerment. This was evidenced by a decrease in employee turnover from more than 70% annually before implementation to less than 10% for 3 consecutive years after implementation. Family satisfaction improved substantially. Steve McAlilly reported a decrease in the number of family complaints about staff from two to four a month before implementation to one complaint per year after implementation.

The implementation was not without its challenges, and changes were made in the implementation process for subsequent Green House sites. The first problem was that there was a high level of doubt and little confidence among middle management, especially the nurses, that the direct care workers would be capable of succeeding in their new roles, and this led to some management turnover. Guide selection and training became a focus of concern as the project unfolded. It became apparent that although the Green House model had called for the Guide to be an LNHA, not all LNHAs have the skills needed to fill this coaching role. It was anticipated that one Guide could manage as many as 10 houses. Three people left their positions as Guide before a lasting Guide was involved. Guides reported feeling unprepared to handle the group dynamics, especially during the storming phase, and they were uncomfortable with the decision-making freedom the teams were given. Most LNHAs had spent their careers in the hierarchical medical model of the traditional nursing home. The transition from this "do as the manager says; the authority figure knows best" model to the collaborative democratic model is a dramatic shift. It requires faith in the potential outcomes and the process and a set of coaching, listening, and communication skills that are not assimilated quickly. The outcomes suggest that careful screening, assessment, and discussion are crucial in selecting a Guide.

Because the educational needs of the Guide were underestimated, training and support were added. This training included the specific skills of coaching, counseling, and group dynamics. Furthermore, a coach was provided for the Guide. This coach provided the Guide with assistance and weekly coaching during the team implementation phases. These changes improved outcomes and helped identify more permanent Guides. It was also found that one Guide could not manage 10 houses, particularly during the teams' storming stage. Therefore, it was important to engage other leaders in the organization to act as assistants to the Guides. CST members have now been educated in this role, and they also receive coaching as they help teams develop.

Phase 1 Green Houses in Tupelo have been operating successfully for more than 3 years. The evaluation results clearly show that the increased job satisfaction, decreased turnover, and high level of job performance are a result of the implementation of the EWTs in the houses.

CHAPTER 6

Effects of Empowered Work Teams in Nursing Homes

There is an urgent need to improve the care provided to nursing home (NH) residents. This is particularly the case when one is concerned for the residents' quality of life and life satisfaction as well as health. A variety of initiatives are under way to address this need. Many of these initiatives propose empowering the direct care workers, with the belief that a change from a hierarchical to an empowering management approach will improve resident care. This study tested whether empowered work teams (EWTs) increase the empowerment of direct care workers and improve performance and job attitudes, as they have in manufacturing settings.

Empirical research to evaluate the effects of EWTs has been done almost exclusively in the manufacturing setting. Much less has focused on the service industry, and little has focused on the long-term care industry (an exception includes Yeatts & Seward, 2000). To reduce this gap in our knowledge base, this chapter reports on the findings from a quasiexperimental study, funded by the Commonwealth Fund, that evaluated the effects of 21 EWTs on employee performance, attitudes, absenteeism, and turnover. More specifically, the following propositions were tested.

Proposition 1: EWTs in NHs positively affect feelings of empowerment, including autonomy, impact, meaningfulness, and competence among the team members.

Proposition 2: EWTs in NHs positively affect the performance of the team members.

Proposition 3: EWTs in NHs have a positive effect on job attitudes, including higher levels of job satisfaction, commitment, and self-esteem and lower burnout.

Proposition 4: EWTs in NHs reduce absenteeism and turnover among team members.

This chapter describes the methods used to evaluate the EWTs, followed by the research findings and their implications.

Much of this chapter was previously published in *The Gerontologist* by Yeatts and Cready (2007).

METHODS

A multimethod, pre–post design was used to examine the effects of EWTs on direct care worker performance and attitude outcomes. Both quantitative and qualitative approaches were used. The quantitative approach used a nonequivalent control, pre–post design (Campbell & Stanley, 1966). EWTs were established in five NHs, and the direct care workers in these NHs (e.g., certified nursing assistants, medical aides, restorative aides) were treated as the experimental group. In general, the activities of the direct care worker EWTs included participating in nurse management decisions related to direct care work, reviewing resident health conditions and making recommendations (e.g., resident would benefit from pureed food), addressing issues provided to them by the nurse management, and dealing with any other issue of direct care worker concern. Five comparable (matching) NHs were selected and their direct care workers treated as controls.

The five NHs selected as the experimental group were chosen from 18 volunteer NHs located in the north Texas region. The criteria used to select the five experimental NHs included the willingness of the nurse management and NH administrator to implement EWTs and the stability of the NH management in terms of job tenure. Additional selection criteria were based on a desire to obtain variation in NH characteristics with regard to size, location (rural versus urban), and ownership (for-profit versus nonprofit). Once the five experimental NHs were selected, an attempt was made to identify comparison NHs of the same size, location, and ownership, and these were invited to participate in the study.

A nonequivalent control group design is a quasiexperimental design; that is, the participants in the experimental and control groups are not randomly placed in the two groups. Instead, the participants are already in the experimental and control groups. An effort was made to select a comparison NH that was as similar as possible to the matching experimental NH. To check for similarity, baseline surveys of direct care workers, nurses, and the residents' family members or significant others were conducted at each of the experimental and comparison NHs. An in-person survey of residents was also undertaken, but the number of residents who were able and willing to be interviewed at both the pre and post time periods was too small for meaningful quantitative analyses. Contributing to the small number was one experimental NH that housed only residents with Alzheimer's disease and its comparison NH that housed a substantial number of such residents. None of these residents could be interviewed.

A comparison of demographic characteristics of the direct care workers, nurses, and family members at baseline for the treatment and comparison groups shows that there were only a few differences (Table 6.1). The experimental group had a slightly lower percentage of female direct care workers (83% versus 92%, respectively). The nurses from the experimental NHs tended to have worked at the NH longer (72 versus 43 months) and were more likely to be non-Hispanic white (79% versus 59%, respectively). When considering the family members or significant others surveyed (henceforth referred to as family members), those from the experimental NHs were slightly more likely to be reporting on a female resident than the family members from the comparison NHs (85% versus 78%, respectively).

Implementation and Description of EWTs

The EWTs consisted of only direct care workers and were implemented in one experimental NH at a time, immediately after their NH's baseline survey. The EWTs were implemented in the first experimental NH in 2002 and in the fifth experimental NH in 2004. Teams typically were organized by shift and by service area (e.g., halls or wings of the NH). In total, 21 EWTs were established in the five experimental NHs. The first NH had roughly 60 residents and three EWTs, the sec-

Table 6.1. Demographic Characteristics of Experimental and Comparison Direct Care Workers, Nurses, and Residents

Demographic Characteristics[a]	Experimental Nursing Homes	Comparison Nursing Homes	Significance Test Results[b]
Nurse Aides			
Mean years of education	12.0	11.7	ns
Percentage female nurse aides	82.9	92.3	.011
Mean age (years)	36.2	37.5	ns
Mean number of children	1.5	1.4	ns
Percentage with difficulty paying bills	42.9	41.9	ns
Mean months at nursing home	42.0	36.7	ns
Race or ethnicity			ns
Percentage non-Hispanic white	51.8	41.8	
Percentage non-Hispanic black	32.3	40.0	
Percentage Hispanic or other	15.9	18.2	
Nurses			
Mean years of education	13.9	14.1	ns
Percentage female nurses	93.6	91.4	ns
Mean age (years)	45.1	44.2	ns
Mean number of children	1.2	1.2	ns
Percentage with difficulty paying bills	18.7	18.8	ns
Mean months at nursing home	72.3	42.7	.004
Race or ethnicity			.026
Percentage non-Hispanic white	79.1	59.4	
Percentage non-Hispanic black	12.8	27.5	
Percentage Hispanic or other	8.1	13.0	
Residents or Family Members and Significant Others			
Resident's education	11.6	11.4	ns
Percentage female residents	84.6	78.0	.052
Age of resident	83	84	ns
Months lived in nursing home	38.3	34.6	ns
Percentage under financial hardship	33.6	31.9	ns
Resident's race			ns
Percentage white	98.7	95.9	
Percentage black	1.0	3.3	
Percentage other	0.3	0.8	

Notes:

[a]Includes direct care workers, nurses, and residents or family members associated with the 10 nursing homes participating in the baseline survey. The number of direct care workers ranged from 314 to 353, nurses from 149 to 164, and residents or family members from 530 to 578, with the variation between characteristics due to missing data.

[b]P values from two-tailed t or chi-square tests; ns indicates that the difference between the experimental and comparison groups is not statistically significant ($p > .05$).

ond 80 residents and five EWTs, the third 100 residents and four EWTs, the fourth 200 residents and seven EWTs, and the fifth 50 residents and two EWTs.

The procedures that were used to implement the direct care worker EWTs were pretested at an earlier date in an NH not included in the current study (see Part III and the Appendix for details on how to implement EWTs in long-term care settings). In short, implementation started with orienting and training direct care workers, nurses, and nurse management. Once staff members were familiar with their respective roles and the expected activities of the EWTs, nurse management began making efforts to involve the EWTs in management decisions related to direct care work. For example, the EWT might be asked to provide revised work procedures for distributing breakfast trays so that residents would get hotter meals than the current procedures allowed, or the EWT might be asked to revise procedures for answering call lights so that less time elapsed before a direct care worker responded to a call light.

At the same time, direct care workers began holding weekly 30-minute meetings (initially with the assistance of the authors, Yeatts and Cready, as team facilitators) and short stand-up meetings during the week as needed. The weekly 30-minute meetings followed a set agenda that included not only issues provided by nurse management but also other areas of focus such as a review of resident health conditions, a review of new residents and their specific needs, and any issues of concern to the direct care workers. Weekly written summaries (i.e., minutes) of each team meeting were provided by the team to nurse management, and any direct care worker recommendations or suggestions regarding their work or the residents typically were provided in these weekly summaries. The nurse management reviewed the team summaries and provided weekly written feedback to each EWT. Feedback typically included responses to any direct care worker questions or concerns.

If nurse management was responding to an EWT-proposed change to the work process (e.g., the process for handing out meal trays), nurse management typically responded in one of several ways. In some cases, the proposed EWT change was approved as submitted and the EWT was asked to begin using the revised procedure. In other cases, the nurse management sent the proposed change back to the team, pointed out some shortcomings of the proposed procedure, and asked the team to resubmit the proposed change with this new information in mind. Once management and the EWT came to an agreement on what would work, the proposed change was implemented.

Short stand-up meetings were used by the EWT to address more immediate concerns handed to them by nurse management. For example, nurse management might call the direct care workers together and ask them to determine the best way for the EWT to get all residents to a planned activity when one of their team members was unexpectedly absent. The nurse manager would then leave, and the direct care workers would discuss the alternatives, make a decision, and implement it.

Although five pairs of NHs were initially selected for the study, one pair had to be dropped. In this pair, EWTs were initially implemented successfully in the experimental NH. However, about 6 months after team implementation, the assistant NH administrator chose to assume the role of EWT facilitator. Subsequently, the recommendations made by the team not only were provided to nurse management but were immediately acted on by the assistant administrator. The nurse management perceived this as usurping their authority; in other words, the direct care workers were going around the nurse management and taking their concerns and suggestions directly to the NH administrator. This empowered the direct care worker teams greatly until the NH administrator left the NH for another position and the assistant NH administrator did likewise about 6 weeks later. The nurse management then chose to discontinue the EWTs, and the new NH administrator, being unfamiliar with the EWTs, followed the recommendations of the nurse management in discontinuing the teams.

In addition, EWTs initially were started among night shift direct care workers, but after experiencing some problems most were eventually discontinued. The primary problems encountered were the small numbers of direct care workers who worked the night shift and the irregular staffing of these direct care workers. In most of the experimental NHs, there were three or fewer night shift direct care workers working in a service area (e.g., one floor of the NH). Furthermore, of these direct care workers only a few were permanent night shift staff; the others worked primarily on the day or evening shifts and occasionally worked on the night shift.

Data Collection

The timing for collection of the post data varied somewhat between NHs depending on the schedules and availability of the NH staffs to participate in the follow-up surveys. On average, there was a 16-month period between Time 1 and Time 2 for the experimental NHs and a 17-month period for the comparison NHs. Previous research has shown that the effects of interventions, such as EWTs, can look promising in the short term of 6 to 12 months (the "honeymoon" effect), with the effects becoming less pronounced over time (Lawler, 1986; Lawler & Mohrman, 1987). Therefore, the 16- to 17-month follow-up was selected in part to avoid such premature conclusions.

The baseline and post data collection included self-administered questionnaires for the direct care workers and nurses and a mail survey of the residents' family members. In most cases, the self-administered questionnaires were distributed by the research team at an all-staff meeting of direct care workers and nurses. Each questionnaire was given a unique number and placed in an envelope addressed to a specific direct care worker or nurse, who was handed the envelope by the researcher. This resulted in each direct care worker having a unique questionnaire number. Once completed, the questionnaires were immediately collected by the research staff. Thus the direct care worker or nurse could fill out the questionnaire without her name on it. Simultaneously, the researchers had a unique number for each direct care worker and nurse that was given to them again at the follow-up survey so that their responses from the second survey could be matched and compared to the first. Direct care workers and nurses who were not in attendance were later approached by a member of the research team and invited to participate. In a few cases, the NH management preferred that the questionnaires not be distributed at all-staff meetings. In these cases, the researchers approached the direct care workers and nurses at their work locations during their work hours and invited them to participate. Not using the all-staff meeting to collect the data did not appear to affect the quality of the data collected or the response rates. For the survey of family members, the NH management typically provided the researchers with a mailing list that consisted of one family member (or significant other) for each NH resident. These people were mailed a questionnaire with an addressed, stamped envelope that was mailed back to the researchers.

The pretest response rates for direct care workers at the experimental and comparison NHs were 84% and 92%, respectively; the response rates for nurses were 84% and 80%, respectively; and the pretest mail response rates for family members were 69% and 52%, respectively. Response rates from the post surveys were similar but generally slightly lower.

Questionnaire Items, Concepts, and Indices

The survey instruments for the direct care workers and nurses asked them to respond to a series of statements by using a five-point Likert-type scale ranging from 1 (*strongly disagree*) to 5 (*strongly agree*). Many of the statements were drawn from a number of existing instruments that measure employee empowerment and the other work-related concepts. These instruments included those developed by Cook and colleagues (Cook, Hepworth, Wall, & Warr, 1979), Hackman and Oldham (1980), Maslach and colleagues (Maslach, Jackson, & Leiter, 1996), McGee and Ford (1987), Quinn and Staines (1979), Spreitzer (1995), and Yeatts and Hyten (1998). Where necessary, statements were modified to reflect the uniqueness of the NH environment. For example, the word *recipients* was replaced by the word *residents* in burnout statements such as "I feel I treat some residents as impersonal objects" (Maslach et al., 1996). When statements could not be found in previous studies, statements were developed and pretested at an NH not included in the study.

The family questionnaire used a five-point Likert-type scale ranging from 1 (*yes, always*) to 5 (*no, never*). These scores were reversed to maintain consistency across the tables; that is, the larger the number (5) the more positive the response (*yes, always*). For the family questionnaire, several questions were taken from a 17-item satisfaction scale presented by Kruzich and colleagues (Kruzich, Clinton, & Kelber, 1992). Additional questions came from an NH satisfaction survey instrument developed jointly by Scripps Gerontology Center and the Margaret Blenkner Research Center (Straker, 2001) and from an instrument developed and presented by Uman Cohen-Mansfield, Ejaz, and Werner (2000). Still other questions were drawn from instruments developed by Bliesmer and Earle (1993), Davis and colleagues (Davis, Sebastian, & Tschetter, 1997), and Kleinsorge and Koenig (1991).

The questionnaire items typically were used to create indices to represent various concepts. The majority of indices consisted of three or more items. For example, the indexed variable for direct care workers' perceptions of global empowerment consisted of 19 statements, including items measuring its dimensions of autonomy (e.g., "The nurse aides decide the procedures for getting residents to the dining room"), competence (e.g., "When a new resident is admitted, I am given all the information I need about the new resident"), and impact or meaningfulness (e.g., "The management staff listens to the suggestions of direct care workers"). On the other hand, the indexed variable for general job satisfaction consisted of only three statements (e.g., "Generally speaking, I am very satisfied with my work"). Furthermore, for two of the concepts from the direct care worker and nurse questionnaires—direct care worker self-reported absenteeism and direct care worker satisfaction with scheduling—only a single statement was used. Four concepts from the family questionnaire—spends time on needs, checks on comfort, satisfaction with the care provided, and satisfaction with staff friendliness—also relied on a single item.

The specific items included in an index were determined after an examination of factor analyses and Cronbach's alpha based on standardized items. Standardized alphas were calculated twice for each concept: once at Time 1 (pretest) and again for Time 2 (posttest). They ranged in size from a low of .50 (autonomy at Time 1) to a high of .90 (nurse perception of direct care worker empowerment, Time 1, and nurse perception of time available for paperwork, Time 1). The majority of direct care worker indices ranged in their standardized alphas from .60 to .85. All the nurse indices ranged between .71 and .90, and the majority of family indices ranged in their standardized alphas from .70 to .85.

To calculate each index, the items for a specific concept were added together, and the resulting sum was divided by the number of items added together. This calculation allowed the index score to remain in the original range of the individual items.

Concepts that were measured from direct care worker questionnaire statements included global empowerment and its dimensions of autonomy, impact or meaningfulness, and competence as well as rating of direct care worker performance, self-esteem, burnout, job satisfaction, satisfaction with scheduling, commitment, intent to quit, and absenteeism. Originally, the questionnaire was designed to measure impact and meaningfulness as two separate concepts. However, a factor analysis and standardized alphas showed that the statements used to measure these concepts actually measured a single concept. Therefore, a single index was created and is referred to as impact or meaningfulness. Direct care worker turnover was measured by determining the percentage of direct care workers working at Time 1 who were still working at the same NH at Time 2. A separate calculation was made for the experimental NHs and for the comparison NHs.

Concepts that were measured from nurse questionnaire statements included

- global direct care worker empowerment;

- direct care worker procedures;

- direct care worker coordination;

- direct care worker cooperation with nurses;

- nurse time to complete paperwork.

Concepts concerning the direct care to residents that were measured from family member questionnaire items included

- spends time on resident needs;

- checks on resident comfort;

- responds to resident complaints;

- listens, talks, and cares for resident.

Other concepts from the family questionnaire included satisfaction with care provided, satisfaction with staff friendliness, residents have choice of bedtime, residents have choice of meal time, and residents have choice of shower time.

Qualitative Approach

The qualitative approach consisted of observations of more than 270 direct care worker team meetings, an examination of weekly team meeting summaries provided by the direct care worker EWTs to nurse management, and an examination of written weekly responses and requests from nurse management to the EWTs. For each EWT, the first 8 to 12 weekly meetings were observed by one of the principal investigators, who also served as facilitators of the first 2 to 4 weekly meetings. It was determined that the 30-minute team meetings provided the most fruitful information about the team's effects because the direct care workers had a block of time available to them to make decisions that affected their work processes and performance, to express their attitudes about their work, and to discuss turnover and absenteeism issues. The times of the weekly meetings typically were established by the teams themselves and usually were scheduled either during the slowest part of the team's shift or during the shift change so that direct care workers from the next shift could join them. Additional meetings were randomly observed roughly once every 3 months for the next 12 months. In most cases, immediately after an observation the observer jotted down a summary of what occurred at the meeting. The notes were organized chronologically. Additionally, copies of the weekly summaries submitted to nurse management by the EWTs were provided to the researchers for the first 12 weeks that the team met and then irregularly thereafter (roughly once every 3 months for 9 additional months). Furthermore, copies of nurse management's written weekly responses to the EWTs each week and any other information they wanted to share with the team were also provided to the researchers for the first 12 weeks and then roughly every 3 months after that for 9 additional months.

Data Analyses

To test the propositions, both the qualitative and quantitative data were analyzed. A review of the qualitative data (observations, EWT weekly summaries, and nurse management weekly written responses) was conducted separately for each proposition. During each review, the data were examined for trends that refuted or supported the proposition. The qualitative findings are presented for each proposition.

For the quantitative analysis, only the responses from direct care workers, nurses, and family members who participated in both the pre and post surveys were included. It was reasoned that changes in the responses of these direct care workers, nurses, and family members, if any, would most accurately reflect any effects of the EWTs.

Several reliability checks of the quantitative data were performed. For three pairs of statements included in the questionnaire for direct care workers, each statement in a pair was identical, or the statements were the same except that one was worded in the opposite direction (positive statement versus negative statement). If the respondent was not consistent in her responses on at least two of the three pairs of questions, her responses were examined for possible coding errors or excessive influence on overall scores. No such respondents were found. In addition, for the multivariate analyses, Mahalanobis distance scores were used to uncover any respondents who were outliers on the variables used. Here again, no respondent was identified as needing to be removed from further analysis.

To examine change between Times 1 and 2, t tests were used for the experimental group and for the comparison group. A t test allows one to determine whether there are differences between two groups beyond what could be expected by chance. To compare the amount of change in the experimental group to the amount of change in the comparison group, t tests were again used: First, a new variable that reflects the difference between Times 1 and 2 was created for each respondent, and this difference was regressed on a dummy variable coded 1 if she was in the experimental group and 0 if she was in the comparison group. The p value associated with the dummy variable coefficient estimate allowed us to determine whether the average change (or difference) across time was significantly different between the experimental and comparison groups. Furthermore, because direct care workers, nurses, and family members were clustered within NHs, p values used were based on standard errors adjusted for this clustering (see StataCorp, 2003, p. 328). Additionally, because the large number of t tests increases the chance of committing a Type 1 error (rejecting the null hypothesis of no difference when it is true), multivariate analysis of variance (MANOVA) was performed. For the MANOVAs, all assumptions were met and appropriate diagnostics were conducted.

FINDINGS

Proposition 1. *EWTs in NHs positively affect feelings of empowerment, including autonomy, impact, meaningfulness, and competence among the team members.* Both the qualitative and quantitative data support this proposition.

Results from Direct Care Workers

Observations of EWT meetings and of direct care workers at their work revealed that

1. The autonomy of the direct care workers within the EWTs increased somewhat because nurse management consulted with the EWTs, sometimes allowed

them to make decisions about their work, and allowed them to work on their own.

2.   The direct care workers became more competent in performing their work as the team meetings allowed them to learn more about their work responsibilities and the preferences and health conditions of residents.

3.   The direct care workers were able to experience the impact of their improved competence as they used their new knowledge to assist residents.

It was less clear from a review of the qualitative observation data whether the EWTs affected the meaningfulness of the work to direct care workers. Generally, it appeared that the direct care workers already held this view, and so the EWTs had little effect.

Although observation notes clearly show that the direct care workers' empowerment was increased, the amount of increase is less clear. Observations revealed that direct care workers were at times given opportunities to make decisions, but these were not routine. This appeared to be due to a perception by management that some decisions had to be made quickly, and so there was no time to consult with the EWTs; nurse management sometimes simply forgot to include the EWTs in decision making; and empowering workers is a different way of thinking that takes time and effort, and so it was almost always easier for nurse management to make decisions without consulting with the direct care worker teams.

Examination of the direct care worker pre (Time 1) and post (Time 2) questionnaire data confirms that there was an increase in empowerment, although the increase was modest (Table 6.2). The direct care workers in the experimental NHs reported higher levels of global empowerment, autonomy, impact or meaningfulness, and competence at Time 2 than Time 1, whereas the direct care workers in the comparison group showed no significant change between time periods. In addition, the differences over time on these measures between the experimental and comparison groups were for the most part significant (Table 6.2, last column).

An explanation for the lack of larger effects on the experimental group may be the higher empowerment expectations of this group at Time 2 than Time 1. At Time 1 they perceived themselves neutral to slightly empowered (3.2 on a 5-point scale). At Time 2 the direct care workers had more knowledge about empowerment and had higher expectations about direct care worker empowerment. Consequently, at Time 2 they still reported themselves as being only slightly more empowered (3.4) even though the qualitative observation data showed that their level of autonomy, competence, and impact had clearly increased.

Results from Nursing Staff

Another means of examining this proposition, while avoiding any contamination issues caused by direct care worker awareness of empowerment at Time 2, is an examination of the nurses' perceptions (Table 6.2, bottom panel). Consistent with Proposition 1, these findings suggest that the EWTs positively affected direct care worker empowerment. The nurses in the experimental group perceived more direct care worker empowerment at Time 2 than Time 1, while the nurses in the comparison group did not perceive any change. Furthermore, in a comparison of the difference over time between the experimental and comparison groups, a significant effect is again found (Table 6.2, last column).

Proposition 2. *EWTs in NHs positively affect the performance of the team members.* This proposition is also supported by both the qualitative and the quantitative data.

Results from Direct Care Workers

The qualitative observation data indicate that the EWTs assisted the direct care workers in becoming more aware of resident health conditions. This reduced the possibility that a resident health problem would go unattended for an extended pe-

Table 6.2. DCWs' and Nurses' Perceptions of DCW Empowerment by Treatment Group (Experimental and Comparison) and Time (1 and 2)

Concept[a]	Time 1 Mean (*N*)	Time 2 Mean (*N*)	Significance of Difference Between Time 1 and Time 2 Within Group[b]	Significance of Difference Between Time 1 and Time 2 Between Groups[c]
DCWs' Perceptions of DCW Empowerment				
Global empowerment				
Experimental	3.2 (49)	3.4 (49)	.021	.021
Comparison	3.4 (43)	3.5 (43)	*ns*	
Autonomy				
Experimental	3.1 (53)	3.3 (53)	.022	.030
Comparison	3.3 (48)	3.3 (48)	*ns*	
Impact or meaningfulness				
Experimental	3.2 (58)	3.4 (58)	.042	.034
Comparison	3.5 (47)	3.5 (47)	*ns*	
Competence				
Experimental	2.8 (60)	2.9 (60)	.015	.090
Comparison	3.1 (46)	3.1 (46)	*ns*	
Nurses' Perceptions of DCW Empowerment				
Global empowerment				
Experimental	3.2 (35)	3.5 (35)	.010	.007
Comparison	3.5 (23)	3.4 (23)	*ns*	

Notes: DCW = direct care worker.

[a]The higher the mean, the more of the characteristic.

[b]For each characteristic, this column reports the *p* value for a one-tailed paired *t* test of the mean difference between Time 1 and Time 2 on the characteristic within a given treatment group. Thus an *ns* in this column indicates that the mean difference between Time 1 and Time 2 on global empowerment within the comparison group is not statistically significant ($p > .05$).

[c]For each characteristic, this column reports the *p* value for a one-tailed independent *t* test of the mean difference between Time 1 and Time 2 on the characteristic between treatment groups; thus an *ns* in this column indicates that the mean difference between Time 1 and Time 2 on the characteristic between the experimental and comparison groups is not statistically significant ($p > .05$). *P* values were generated by regressing the difference between Time 1 and Time 2 for DCWs or nurses on a dummy variable coded 1 if the DCW or nurse worked in an experimental nursing home and coded 0 otherwise, and they were based on standard errors adjusted for the clustering of DCWs or nurses in facility (see StataCorp, 2003, p. 328).

riod of time and increased the possibility that proper health care would be provided. For example, in one team meeting, one of the direct care workers informed the others that Ms. Smith preferred to be taken to the toilet rather than using a bedpan. The response from another direct care worker was that Ms. Smith had recently had a hip replacement and should not get out of bed. This important bit of information may have saved Ms. Smith a serious reinjury of her hip because all the direct care workers quickly agreed that Ms. Smith should not get out of bed in the future until the nurses and doctor found the hip to be in a condition to do so.

Second, the EWTs provided direct care workers with information about the special care needs, uniqueness, and preferences of residents. For example, a direct care worker might report in a team meeting that a particular resident prefers using a particular bathroom. In another case a direct care worker reported having difficulty turning Mr. Jones in bed without him becoming combative. Another direct care worker responded by explaining that Mr. Jones was willing to be turned as long as he was slid up against the wall before being turned.

Third, team meetings provided an opportunity for direct care workers to have frank discussions about any questionable behaviors of other direct care workers. Such discussions provided the opportunity to clarify one's actions. Clarification often resulted in reduced frustration and animosity among direct care workers and an increased willingness to cooperate and coordinate the care provided to residents. In some cases, poor-performing direct care workers were confronted by the EWT and provided instruction by the team on how to improve their performance. This instruction was also found to be valuable for new direct care workers. When a direct care worker was repeatedly performing at a low level, it was sometimes brought up in a team meeting. Team members would describe why the performance was poor and clarify what should be done to improve the performance. This sometimes resulted in the poor performer learning from the team and improving. In extreme cases, if the poor performer was unreceptive to constructive criticism, the EWT contributed to the direct care worker being fired by reporting the poor performance to nurse management on multiple occasions.

Fourth, new work procedures appeared to be carried out more willingly by direct care workers and to remain a part of their work routine longer when the direct care workers participated in creating the new procedures. For example, in one NH three pairs of direct care workers served three halls. One of the pairs of direct care workers was taking longer to get the work done, so nurse management suggested that the direct care workers from the other two halls take turns assisting those on the third hall. The direct care workers were unhappy with this solution because they believed that the slower pair of direct care workers was simply not putting in enough effort. After some back and forth discussion with the direct care workers, the director of nursing (DON) allowed the direct care workers to implement their own solution, which was for the pairs of direct care workers to take turns working on the third hall. The result of this solution was that the direct care workers came to realize that the third hall was indeed more difficult to serve. Consequently, they no longer resented having to help out the direct care workers on this third hall. A complete list of the positive effects found from the qualitative data is provided in Exhibit 6A.

The qualitative observation data also provided evidence that the EWTs may have had some negative effects on resident care because direct care workers were pulled away from direct resident care for 30 minutes while they attended a weekly EWT meeting. In all experimental NHs, the direct care workers had difficulty finding time for their team meetings. The job of direct care workers is difficult; often they do not have time to do all that needs to be done and consequently must choose which tasks will get done and which will not. The team meetings reduced the time available to provide resident care by at least 30 minutes each week.

In addition, the positive effects of the EWTs on performance appeared to be experienced in a repeating cycle from more effect on performance to less effect and back again. When the EWT had an issue to address that was perceived to be important to the NH management or residents or to the direct care workers themselves, a high level of energy and enthusiasm was applied to the issue. When there were no burning issues of interest or DON-requested problems to be solved during the EWT meetings, the direct care workers showed less enthusiasm, and thus it appeared that less was accomplished.

The quantitative survey data also support the performance proposition. For example, when experimental group direct care workers were queried about the EWTs in the post questionnaire, the majority of them agreed or strongly agreed that the EWTs allow them to learn from each other (58%) and learn what the residents like and dislike (59%), with 22% and 19% disagreeing or strongly disagreeing, respectively (Table 6.3). Similarly, the majority of nurses reported that the EWTs provide new ideas that are helpful (57%) and create helpful ways of doing their work (59%), with 11% and 9% disagreeing or strongly disagreeing, respectively. Sixty percent of the direct care workers disagreed with the statement "We should stop using teams," and only 15% agreed or strongly agreed. Similarly, 63% of the nurses responded negatively to the suggestion of stopping teams, with 11% responding positively. Neutral responses to these statements included new direct care workers and nurses who were not yet familiar with the effects or lack of effects of the EWTs.

Results from Nursing Staff

An examination of the pre (Time 1) and post (Time 2) data from nurse questionnaires shows similar findings, whereas the direct care worker data provide less support (Table 6.4, first two panels). Although direct care workers in the experimental NHs reported significantly higher performance at Time 2 than Time 1, the increase was slight (3.7 versus 3.6) and not significantly different from the trend of no change reported by direct care workers in the comparison NHs. On the other hand, the significant improvements found over time on direct care worker performance measures among the nurses in the experimental NHs were both larger and, on the whole, significantly different from the lack of improvement on these measures reported by nurses in the comparison NHs (Table 6.4, second panel, last

EXHIBIT 6A.

Positive Effects of Empowered Work Teams Found from Qualitative Data

- *There is less likelihood that a resident health problem will go unattended for an extended period.* Team meetings include a review of residents who appear to be developing a health problem (e.g., skin breakdown). These health problems are then included in the team's weekly notes to nurse management.

- *Direct care workers are better informed about the health conditions of the residents.* This includes skin conditions, recent eating habits, any recent accidents, and behavioral problems. Such information sometimes is passed to the team by nurses and at other times by team members who notice a health condition and report it to the team. Direct care workers are able to provide better care to residents as a result of this improved information from nurses and other direct care workers.

- *Direct care workers are more willing to assist one another when caring for residents.* Team meetings provide an opportunity for direct care workers to discuss any questionable behaviors by other direct care workers. Such discussions provide the opportunity to clarify one's actions. Clarification often reduces animosity between direct care workers and increases willingness to support one another when caring for residents.

- *Poor-performing direct care workers are confronted by the team.* In some cases, a team confronts a direct care worker who is not performing her duties very well (e.g., leaving incontinent residents wet for hours at a time). The team clarifies for the direct care worker what the problems are and typically expresses the concern that they cause. When this occurs, the poor-performing direct care worker has an opportunity to explain her performance (e.g., why she is unable to assist incontinent residents sooner), and the other direct care workers have an opportunity to provide suggestions about how the performance can be improved (e.g., what the direct care worker can do that will allow her to assist the incontinent residents in a more timely manner). This results in the poor performer accepting that her current performance is not adequate and learning from the team what she needs to do in order to improve.

- *Direct care workers learn from one another how to perform their daily tasks better.* For example, if a direct care worker is slow at performing a particular task, other direct care workers question her about the procedures she is following and provide suggestions about how she can revise her work procedures to get her work done more quickly.

- *New direct care workers learn quickly about resident preferences and the daily procedures followed to care for them.* Team meetings typically include a discussion of resident preferences (e.g., who likes to attend bingo) and often include a discussion of the procedures followed to complete a particular task (e.g., handing out meal trays while answering call lights).

- *Direct care workers learn about the special care needs and unique traits of residents.* For example, a direct care worker reports in a team meeting that a particular resident prefers using a particular bathroom. On another occasion a direct care worker reports that a

EXHIBIT 6A. *(continued)*

particular resident is combative when being turned in bed, then learns from another that the resident is willing to be turned if she is slid up against the wall first.

- *Direct care workers identify the most efficient procedures for carrying out a particular task.* Direct care workers are more knowledgeable about the residents and the work needed to assist them than anyone else in the nursing home. Consequently, they are better able to identify the procedures that can satisfy the need to get a task completed in a timely manner and also satisfy the residents' preferences.

- *Direct care workers learn the preferences of other direct care workers and distribute the work so that they are doing those things they prefer.* For example, if one direct care worker prefers answering call lights and another prefers assisting residents with eating, they can distribute their work so that each is doing what she prefers.

- *Solutions to problems are carried out more willingly by direct care workers* and are more likely to become a regular part of the work day because the direct care workers have been involved in identifying the solution and subsequently have identified one that they are willing to carry out and feel a commitment to.

- *Direct care workers learn the best matches between workers and residents.* Residents are more satisfied with their care because they are being cared for by the person they prefer. This might apply to particular caring activities such as bathing or to more general care activities.

- *Absenteeism may be reduced.* Direct care workers have the time to discuss absenteeism issues and the advantages that occur when everyone comes to work each day. In such discussions, direct care workers learn about the problems they are causing by their absence and subsequently make more of an effort to be at work. Furthermore, other direct care workers learn why someone needs to be absent and may offer help so the absence can be avoided.

---

column). The nurses from the experimental NHs rated the direct care worker procedures used to do the work at a higher level at Time 2 than Time 1 (4.1 versus 3.8), whereas the comparison group of nurses showed no difference. Similar results were observed for nurse ratings of direct care worker coordination. A MANOVA (not shown) that included all the nurse variables confirmed these findings; specifically, the treatment group effect was significant ($p = .035$), suggesting, again, that the EWTs improved nurses' perceptions of direct care worker performance. Why the nurses perceived higher performance at Time 2 and the direct care workers did not is difficult to determine. Perhaps the direct care workers did not perceive a change in performance because of an inability to see the forest for the trees. That is, it may have been difficult for the direct care workers to recognize the higher performance because of their daily involvement in the teams.

It is interesting to note that the teams appeared to have positive effects on nurse performance. The nurses from the experimental NHs reported more time to complete their paperwork at Time 2 than Time 1 (2.9 versus 2.4), a trend that was marginally different ($p = .068$) from the no change between time periods reported by the comparison nurses.

Results from Resident Families

Family member pre and post responses indicated that some measures of direct care worker performance were affected by the EWTs whereas others were not. Three of four measures of direct care were found to be slightly higher at Time 2 than Time 1 for the experimental group, whereas no differences were found for the comparison group (Table 6.4, third panel). The three measures that improved were "spends time on resident needs" (4.2 versus 4.4), "checks on resident comfort" (4.2 versus 4.4), and "staff listens, talks, and cares" (4.4 versus 4.5). However, when in a comparison of the changes on these measures between the experimental and comparison groups, the only significant difference was for "staff listens, talks, and cares" (Table 6.4, third panel, last column). The treatment group effect in a MANOVA (not shown), including all four direct care variables, was not significant. Furthermore, an examination of two additional performance measures, "satisfaction with care" and "satisfaction with staff friendliness," showed no differences between the experimental and comparison groups (Table 6.4, fourth panel).

Family members were also asked whether residents were given an opportunity to make choices about the services provided (Table 6.4, fifth panel). Family mem-

Table 6.3. DCW and Nurse Evaluations of Empowered Work Teams

Statements Provided to DCWs and Nurses	% Disagree or Strongly Disagree	% Neutral	% Agree or Strongly Agree
DCW Responses			
In team meetings:			
DCWs learn from each other.	22	20	58
DCWs discuss how the work should be done.	20	23	57
DCWs learn what residents like and don't like.	19	22	59
The team leader makes sure everyone participates.	16	22	62
My team leader makes all the decisions for my team.	59	28	14
We should stop using teams.	60	25	15
Nurse Responses			
DCW team members:			
Provide new ideas that are helpful.	11	32	57
Create helpful ways of doing their work.	9	32	59
Provide solutions to problems.	11	42	47
The nursing home should continue to encourage DCW teams.	11	18	70
The DCW teams have been helpful to me.	14	29	57
Allowing DCWs to make decisions about their work improves resident care.	5	17	78
DCW teams do *not* work well in this nursing home.	63	26	11

Notes: DCW = direct care worker.

Includes all DCWs working in empowered work teams and all nurses at the four experimental nursing homes. The number of DCW respondents ranged from 155 to 159 and nurses from 77 to 80, with the variation between items due to missing data.

Table 6.4. DCWs', Nurses', and Family Members' Perceptions by Treatment Group (Experimental and Comparison) and Time (1 and 2)

Concept[a]	Time 1 Mean (N)	Time 2 Mean (N)	Significance of Difference Between Time 1 and Time 2 Within Group[b]	Significance of Difference Between Time 1 and Time 2 Between Groups[c]
DCWs' Perceptions of DCW Performance				
DCW performance				
Experimental	3.6 (64)	3.7 (64)	.022	ns
Comparison	3.8 (49)	3.9 (49)	ns	
Nurses' Perceptions of DCW Performance				
DCW procedures				
Experimental	3.8 (37)	4.1 (37)	.001	.024[d]
Comparison	3.8 (25)	3.8 (25)	ns	
DCW coordination				
Experimental	3.5 (37)	3.8 (37)	.016	.004[d]
Comparison	3.6 (25)	3.7 (25)	ns	
DCW cooperation with nurses				
Experimental	3.8 (36)	4.0 (36)	.037	ns[d]
Comparison	3.8 (25)	3.9 (25)	ns	
Adequate time to complete nurse paperwork				
Experimental	2.4 (37)	2.9 (37)	.002	.068[d]
Comparison	2.6 (26)	2.7 (26)	ns	
Family Members' Perceptions of Direct Care Provided to Residents				
Spends time on resident needs				
Experimental	4.2 (123)	4.4 (123)	.005	ns[e]
Comparison	4.0 (47)	4.1 (47)	ns	
Checks on resident comfort				
Experimental	4.2 (118)	4.4 (118)	.029	ns[e]
Comparison	4.0 (47)	4.1 (47)	ns	
Responds to complaints				
Experimental	4.0 (70)	4.1 (70)	ns	ns[e]
Comparison	3.9 (35)	3.9 (35)	ns	
Staff listens, talks, cares				
Experimental	4.4 (114)	4.5 (114)	.018	.054[e]
Comparison	4.3 (46)	4.2 (46)	ns	
Family Members' Satisfaction with Care and Staff of NH				
Satisfaction with care provided				
Experimental	4.6 (121)	4.6 (121)	ns	ns
Comparison	4.4 (43)	4.6 (43)	.042	
Satisfaction with staff friendliness				
Experimental	4.6 (121)	4.7 (121)	ns	ns
Comparison	4.4 (44)	4.6 (44)	ns	
Family Members' Perceptions of Choices Available to Residents				
When to go to bed or get up				
Experimental	3.8 (74)	3.8 (74)	ns	.028[d]
Comparison	4.0 (32)	3.6 (32)	.008	
When to eat a meal				
Experimental	2.5 (75)	2.8 (75)	.014	.007[d]
Comparison	3.3 (32)	2.8 (32)	.004	

(continued)

Table 6.4.   *(continued)*

Concept[a]	Time 1 Mean (*N*)	Time 2 Mean (*N*)	Significance of Difference Between Time 1 and Time 2 Within Group[b]	Significance of Difference Between Time 1 and Time 2 Between Groups[c]
Family Members' Perceptions of Choices Available to Residents *continued*				
When to shower				
Experimental	2.6 (74)	2.9 (74)	.013	.001[d]
Comparison	2.8 (31)	2.4 (31)	.008	
DCW Job Attitudes				
Self-esteem				
Experimental	4.1 (58)	4.1 (58)	*ns*	*ns*[e]
Comparison	4.2 (48)	4.2 (48)	*ns*	
Burnout				
Experimental	2.3 (58)	2.2 (58)	*ns*	*ns*[e]
Comparison	2.2 (41)	2.2 (41)	*ns*	
General job satisfaction				
Experimental	4.1 (63)	4.0 (63)	*ns*	*ns*[e]
Comparison	4.0 (49)	3.9 (49)	*ns*	
Satisfaction with scheduling				
Experimental	3.2 (57)	3.6 (57)	.034	.028[e]
Comparison	3.2 (50)	3.1 (50)	*ns*	
Commitment				
Experimental	4.0 (61)	4.0 (61)	*ns*	*ns*[e]
Comparison	4.2 (46)	3.9 (46)	.026	
Intent to quit				
Experimental	1.9 (60)	2.0 (60)	*ns*	*ns*[e]
Comparison	2.0 (47)	2.1 (47)	*ns*	
DCW Absenteeism and Turnover				
Self-reported absenteeism				
Experimental	1.2 (48)	1.3 (48)	*ns*	*ns*
Comparison	1.3 (35)	1.6 (35)	.023	
Turnover (percentage no longer working)[f]				
Experimental		36.8% (149)		.014
Comparison		50.8% (179)		

Notes: DCW = direct care worker; NH = nursing home.

[a] The higher the mean, the more of the characteristic.

[b] For each characteristic, this column reports the *p* value for a one-tailed paired *t* test of the mean difference between Time 1 and Time 2 on the characteristic within a given treatment group. Thus *ns* in this column indicates that the mean difference between Time 1 and Time 2 on DCWs' perceptions of DCW performance within the comparison group is not statistically significant ($p > .05$).

[c] For each characteristic, this column reports the *p* value for a one-tailed independent *t* test of the mean difference between Time 1 and Time 2 on the characteristic between treatment groups. Thus *ns* in this column indicates that the mean difference between Time 1 and Time 2 on DCWs' perceptions of DCW performance between the experimental and comparison groups is not statistically significant ($p > .05$). *P* values were generated by regressing the difference between Time 1 and Time 2 for DCWs or nurses on a dummy variable coded 1 if the DCW or nurse worked in an experimental NH and coded 0 otherwise, and they were based on standard errors adjusted for the clustering of DCWs or nurses in the facility (see StataCorp, 2003, p. 328).

[d] The treatment group effect of a MANOVA including this variable and all other variables in this domain (e.g., nurse perceptions of DCW performance) was statistically significant ($p > .05$).

[e] The treatment group effect of a MANOVA including this variable and all other variables in this domain was not statistically significant ($p > .05$).

[f] Turnover was calculated separately for each treatment group as the percentage of DCWs who were working at Time 1 who were no longer working at the same NH at Time 2. Accordingly, the *p* value reported for this variable is from a chi-square test.

bers from the experimental NHs reported a significantly higher level of choice at Time 2 than Time 1 regarding "when to eat" (2.8 versus 2.5) and "when to shower" (2.9 versus 2.6). Family members from the comparison NHs reported lower levels of choice at Time 2 than Time 1 on these and the "when to sleep" variables. The trend of more choice in the experimental group was significantly different from the trend of less choice in the comparison group (Table 6.4, fifth panel, last column). The result of a MANOVA that included the three choice variables confirms the findings ($p = .005$). It is reasonable to suspect that the increased choices available to residents in the experimental NHs were the result of the direct care workers having better knowledge of the residents' preferences, as noted from the qualitative observation data.

> **Proposition 3.** *EWTs in NHs have a positive effect on job attitudes, including higher levels of job satisfaction, commitment, and self-esteem and lower burnout.* This proposition is partially supported by qualitative data and unsupported by the quantitative data.

Results from Direct Care Workers

In support of Proposition 3 were observation data that showed that direct care workers were able to distribute the work so that they were more likely to do the kinds of tasks they preferred and serve the particular residents they most enjoyed. For example, if one direct care worker preferred answering call lights and another preferred assisting residents with eating, the direct care workers sometimes were able to distribute their work so that each was doing what she preferred. Similarly, direct care workers sometimes were able to distribute the specific residents according to who preferred serving whom or to share equally in serving a resident whom no one wanted to serve.

On the other hand, observations of EWT meetings suggested that EWTs also have the potential to foster some negative attitudes. Some direct care workers complained that the 30-minute weekly meetings kept them from completing their work on time. In other cases, when team meetings were held before or after a direct care worker's shift, some direct care workers complained that they could not get to work early for the meetings or stay late for the meetings because of other obligations, such as taking a spouse to work or picking up children from school. Still other direct care workers complained about team members who disrupted team meetings by repeatedly bringing up an issue or personal problem that had already been addressed. Finally, direct care workers generally became dissatisfied in cases when a DON neglected to read and respond to the direct care workers' weekly team notes.

Similarly, in general the quantitative survey data did not support the proposition that EWTs have a positive effect on job attitudes. The direct care workers in the experimental NHs and the comparison NHs reported the same levels of general job satisfaction, burnout, and self-esteem at Time 1 and Time 2 (Table 6.4, sixth panel). In one exception the experimental group reported higher satisfaction with scheduling at Time 2 than Time 1, whereas no difference was found among the comparison direct care workers. It is reasonable to suspect that this was the result of the EWTs' ability to influence scheduling decisions. In another exception, the comparison group reported lower commitment at Time 2 than at Time 1, whereas the experimental group showed no change. However, neither the results of *t* tests comparing differences over time between the experimental and the comparison groups (Table 6.4, sixth panel, last column) nor the results of a MANOVA including all the job attitude variables (not shown) were statistically significant.

It is important to note that the lack of effect by EWTs on a direct care worker's job attitudes does not mean that an employee's feelings of empowerment have no effect. In fact, as shown in Chapter 7, direct care worker feelings of empowerment had large impacts on job attitudes.

Proposition 4. *EWTs in NHs reduce absenteeism and turnover among team members.* The proposition is partially supported in this analysis and more closely examined in Chapter 7, where clear positive effects are shown.

Results from Direct Care Workers

The qualitative observation data showed that during team meetings, direct care workers sometimes discussed the problems absenteeism causes. This appeared to help those who were routinely absent to better understand the effects their absences were having on the other direct care workers and appeared to result in greater efforts to be at work. In some cases, direct care workers would report to the team that they were going to be absent and then another would try to help them avoid the absence. For example, in one case a direct care worker reported that she would be absent the next day because her babysitter was not going to be available. A second direct care worker noted that her babysitter would not mind having additional children and that the first direct care worker could leave her kids with this babysitter. This resulted in the direct care worker avoiding being absent.

When considering turnover, the observation data again suggest some positive effects of EWTs. On several occasions during EWT meetings, a direct care worker would comment that she would prefer to stay at the NH because the EWTs seemed to be helping, and other NHs in the local area lacked such teams.

The observation data also uncovered some negative effects on turnover. If a direct care worker was absent routinely, she sometimes spoke of the need to quit because of her inability to avoid absences and its negative effects on the other direct care workers. In other cases, the EWT made an effort to have a direct care worker fired. This was found to occur when the direct care worker was not getting the work done and it was having negative effects on resident care (e.g., when a direct care worker routinely allowed residents to sit in soiled, wet clothing for long periods of time rather than promptly changing the clothing).

In the quantitative survey data, no differences were found in self-reported absenteeism between Time 1 and Time 2 for those in the experimental NHs (Table 6.4, bottom panel). Interestingly, self-reported absenteeism had a statistically significant increase in the comparison group (1.3 versus 1.6). However, although this increase in the comparison NHs seems to suggest that EWTs may help prevent absenteeism, it was not large enough to be significantly different from the stable trend observed for the experimental group (Table 6.4, bottom panel, last column).

On the other hand, direct care workers in experimental NHs were significantly less likely to quit or be terminated (Table 6.4, bottom panel, last column). Only 37% of the direct care workers who were working in the experimental NHs at Time 1 were not working in these same NHs at Time 2. In contrast, at the comparison NHs, 51% were no longer working at the same NHs. However, this difference must be viewed cautiously because the average length of time between Time 1 and Time 2 was a month longer for the comparison NHs, and consequently there was an additional month for direct care workers to quit. (Chapter 7 provides a more in-depth analysis of the effects of EWTs on turnover. This analysis shows that, controlling for the length of time between the Time 1 and Time 2 surveys, EWTs significantly reduced turnover.)

DISCUSSION

The implementation of the direct care worker EWTs began with a pilot project in a single NH, with the subsequent establishment of 21 EWTs in five NHs in the north central Texas region. The process of implementing the EWTs was a learning experience for the research team, so implementation in the fifth experimental NH occurred more quickly and easily than in the first NH. Therefore, the study's results reflect both the effects of the EWTs and the authors' improving EWT implementation skills. The authors also discovered that the size of the NH has a significant impact on the ease of implementation. An NH of 200 residents can have 12 or more EWTs—more than a single DON can monitor, necessitating significant involvement of multiple team facilitators as the teams are getting under way and many more nurse managers to work with and respond to the teams.

The generalizability of the study's findings is also affected by two other substantive limitations. First, because the study is based on a quasiexperimental design conducted in a single region of the United States, its findings may not apply to all NHs. Participating NHs volunteered to join the study and therefore may be somewhat different from the typical NH. Direct care workers, nurses, and family members were not randomly assigned to one NH or another, allowing for the possibility of differences between the groups beyond those already identified (Table 6.1). And because the NHs are all located in north Texas, findings may be influenced by the uniqueness of the location itself. Second, the analytical approach results in the exclusion of missing data; only those who were present at both Time 1 and Time 2 were included in the analyses. Unfortunately, the authors were unable to survey the direct care workers, nurses, and family members who were missing at Time 2 to obtain their attitudes. It is possible that the EWTs had a different effect on those who left the NH before the second survey. Furthermore, it is reasonable to expect that there were baseline differences between those who chose to leave the NHs before Time 2 and those who stayed. A thorough analysis of these data is reported in Chapter 7.

Given these limitations, the qualitative observation data suggest, in general, that the EWTs had positive effects on direct care worker empowerment and performance, possibly positive effects on absenteeism and turnover, and mixed effects on job attitudes. Direct care workers were more empowered after working in EWTs because they were given new decision-making responsibilities, grew in competence at decision making, and experienced more positive impacts from their efforts. However, it was also observed that although nurse management did involve the EWTs in decision making, this involvement could have been more routine.

The EWTs had positive impacts on direct care workers' performance by allowing them to become more aware of resident health conditions, providing them with more information on the special care needs of residents, giving them the opportunity to question the poor performance of negligent team members, and giving them the time needed to clear up misinformation and communication. Furthermore, the team members were more willing to carry out decisions that they participated in making. On the other hand, the observation data also suggest some negative effects on performance, related to the time spent in the meetings, which pulled direct care workers away from their direct care duties. Moreover, the data also suggest that if nurse management had been more consistent in their weekly communications and feedback to the teams, the positive effects of the EWTs on direct care worker performance probably would have been larger.

It appears that team meetings may have reduced absenteeism and turnover. In some cases team members were able to help another avoid an absence once her circumstances had been brought up during team meeting discussions. And some team members who particularly liked the EWTs commented that the EWTs were an important feature of the NH not offered by other facilities.

Mixed results were found from the qualitative observation data with regard to work attitudes. In some cases, positive effects were apparent where direct care workers were given more opportunity to control who did what during the day and who served which residents. This allowed them to do the kinds of work they preferred. However, on the negative side, direct care workers sometimes expressed frustration at having to rush their direct care duties in order to attend the team meetings. And when meetings were scheduled before or after the direct care workers' shifts, some experienced tension because of other responsibilities outside work that conflicted with the meeting times (see Chapter 7 for an in-depth analysis examining the effects of feelings of empowerment on job attitudes).

The quantitative survey data also show statistically significant positive effects of the EWTs on direct care worker empowerment and performance, although the substantive effects were small. No effects were found on job attitudes or self-reported absenteeism. In addition, although the quantitative survey data showed no effect of the EWTs on direct care workers' intent to quit, there is some evidence that turnover itself may have decreased, and this is confirmed in further analysis of direct care worker turnover provided in Chapter 7.

IMPLICATIONS

The qualitative and quantitative data suggest that EWTs can have positive effects on direct care worker empowerment and performance. This suggests that NH managers looking to improve resident care should consider implementing EWTs. The quantitative data showed no effects from the EWTs on job attitudes, whereas the qualitative data suggest that EWTs may have positive effects when a variety of organizational and management conditions are met. For example, the EWTs did not have positive effects when the scheduling of team meetings was at an undesirable time for the direct care workers, or when they were pulled away from providing direct care of their residents to attend an EWT meeting without having someone to cover for them. Similarly, if nurse management did not provide routine procedures for involving the direct care workers in decision making, or if nurse management did not respond routinely to the notes taken at EWT meetings, then the direct care workers displayed less satisfaction with the EWTs. This suggests that NH managers seeking to improve the job attitudes of their direct care workers should not turn to EWTs for this unless they are willing to implement the appropriate organizational and management conditions along with the EWTs themselves. Of course, these implications should not be confused with empowering workers on an individual level. Chapter 7 shows a large positive relationship between direct care workers' feelings of empowerment and job attitudes.

The qualitative and quantitative data on absenteeism and turnover are not complete enough to make sound recommendations. Some of the data suggest that turnover may be reduced by the use of EWTs, but these data are not complete. Chapter 7 investigates this relationship further and does show a clear effect of EWTs on turnover.

For NH administrators and nurse managers who want to implement EWTs, Part III and the Appendix describe what steps to follow and what should be included in staff training. Success will depend greatly on nurse managers' understanding of what is involved and what they will be responsible for doing and on their desire to create and support EWTs. Furthermore, it is important that the direct care workers be given the opportunity to learn how to work together in a team meeting, to make mistakes, and to routinely contribute to the management decisions made about their work.

CHAPTER 7

Effects of Empowerment on Direct Care Worker Performance, Attitudes, and Turnover

The empowerment of direct care workers is a multifaceted concept (Thomas & Velthouse, 1990). Although having autonomy in decision making is a major component of empowerment, it is not the only one. Other components include impact or meaning and competence. That is, in addition to making decisions about their work, empowered direct care workers also believe that their work is important in that it has meaningful effects, and they believe that they are well trained and competent to do the work (Ford & Fottler, 1995; Kirkman & Rosen, 1999; Spreitzer, 1995; Thomas & Velthouse, 1990).

This chapter looks more closely at how various aspects of empowerment influence the attitudes and performance of direct care workers and whether these feelings affect their commitment to stay on the job.

EFFECTS OF EMPOWERMENT ON STAFF TURNOVER

Castle, Engberg, Anderson, and Men (2007) investigated the relationship between turnover, job satisfaction, and intent to leave the job among 1,779 direct care workers from nursing homes (NHs) in five states. Although they did not explicitly include a measure of empowerment as a predictor, two of their job satisfaction subscales are reasonable proxies for two of the empowerment dimensions. The training subscale measures direct care workers' perceptions of their preparation for their job or competence, and the work content subscale, which includes direct care workers' perceptions of how much they influence residents' lives, captures impact or meaning (Castle et al., 2007, pp. 196, 199). Autonomy in decision making was not measured. They found that both high overall job satisfaction and high training satisfaction are associated with less intent to leave the job and low turnover, controlling for the effects of other worker and facility characteristics. They also found that although high work content satisfaction was not associated with intent to leave the job, it was associated with low turnover. Interestingly, they found that only one measure of intent to leave—searching for a job—was associated with actually leaving the job (i.e., turnover) 1 year later.

A number of other studies have also focused on intent to quit or commitment among direct care workers. Measures of direct care worker empowerment in these studies vary, but only one of the studies captures all three empowerment dimensions.

In a bivariate analysis, Caudill and Patrick (1991–1992) found that less empowered direct care workers on the autonomy and competence dimensions were more likely to be thinking about leaving their job. These direct care workers felt that they did not have input into the planning of resident care and believed that they were not free to criticize or change policy or procedures in their NH. They also reported attending fewer in-service training programs and tended to view their skills less favorably. Similarly, another bivariate analysis examined the direct care workers' attitudes toward the job process, measured as "attitudes toward the adequacy of the material, information, and human resources necessary for the job, and the extent to which [direct care workers] believe they have sufficient authority to do their job well." They found this to be associated with commitment to the NH (Grau, Chandler, Burton, & Kolditz, 1991, p. 51).

In a multivariate analysis, Parsons, Simmons, Penn, and Furlough (2003) found that direct care workers who were not satisfied with their "job-related personal and professional growth and involvement in decisions on the job" were less satisfied with their job and more likely to be planning to look for another one (p. 56). Dissatisfaction with management's efforts to keep direct care workers informed had similar effects.

The purpose of this section is to further examine factors affecting direct care worker turnover, with primary attention given to the effects of empowerment and empowered work teams (EWTs). In particular, we address the following question: *Are direct care workers less likely to leave their NH if they are working in EWTs?*

Methods

The data used for the analyses and subsequent results reported in this chapter are taken from the study to examine the effects of EWTs described in Chapter 6. For this section the primary outcome of interest is turnover. This variable was coded 1 if a direct care worker was no longer employed by the NH at follow-up and coded 0 otherwise. At follow-up, 50% of the direct care workers in our sample were no longer employed by their baseline NH.

Demographic and Job Characteristics

Table 7.1 lists all the variables drawn from the baseline survey. Included among them are various demographic and job characteristics of the direct care workers. Race or ethnicity is measured by a single dummy variable, coded 1 for non-Hispanic whites and 0 for all other races and ethnicities. Three categories of education are represented by two dummy variables. The first is coded 1 for direct care workers with less than a 12th-grade education and 0 otherwise. The second is coded 1 for direct care workers with some college or more and 0 otherwise. Direct care workers having a 12th-grade education, high school diploma, or GED are coded 0 for both categories and serve as the omitted or reference group. Like race or ethnicity, having at least one child in the home, financial strain, and primary job responsibility are represented with dummy variables, coded 1 for direct care workers having at least one child in the home, for those finding it always or usually difficult to pay their bills, and for those with primarily noncertified nursing assistant (CNA) responsibilities, such as administering medications and providing restorative therapies. Employment at the NH ranges from 0 to 120 months or more.

As Table 7.1 shows, 44% of direct care workers in the sample were non-Hispanic white, and only about 27% had attended college. Nearly one half (45%) found it always or usually difficult to pay their bills, and 64% had at least one child at home. An overwhelming majority of direct care workers were routinely engaged in CNA tasks, with only 10% of the direct care workers indicating that their primary responsibility was administering medications, providing restorative therapies, or other non-CNA tasks. The average direct care worker had been employed by his or her NH nearly 3 years (M = 34.8 months); the actual length of service varied from a few weeks to several decades (SD = 38.2 months).

Logistic regression was used for the analysis because the dependent variable, turnover (i.e., direct care workers' status of employment at the time of the follow-up survey), is binary. We estimated a set of seven hierarchical models to assess mediating effects of various work-related attitudes (Table 7.2). Dummy variables, one for each of the 11 NHs where the direct care workers worked, were included in six of the seven models to control for the uniqueness of the individual NHs. In the final, seventh model the dummy variables were not included because the variable "EWTs organized within NHs" is a dummy variable that represented the uniqueness of the NHs in two groups: those with EWTs and those without EWTs. Thus,

Table 7.1.   Sample Characteristics at Baseline

Variable	% or M (SD)	Number of Items[a]	Cronbach's Alpha
Demographic Characteristics			
Non-Hispanic white	44.0%		
Less than 12th grade	24.8%		
Some college or more	27.2%		
At least one child at home	64.4%		
Difficulty paying bills	45.3%		
Job Characteristics			
Medical or restorative aide	10.4%		
Months employed at NH	34.8 (38.2)		
Perceptions of Work Environment[a]			
Adequate DCW staffing	2.8 (1.0)	3	.781
Treated fairly	2.5 (0.8)	5	.757
Can trust other DCWs	4.0 (0.9)	1	
Close friend at NH	43.6%		
Empowerment	3.3 (0.5)	19	.836
Work-Related Attitudes			
Emotional exhaustion	2.6 (0.9)	4	.760
Job satisfaction	3.8 (0.8)	3	.773
Intent to quit job at NH	2.3 (1.0)	3	.754
Commitment to NH	3.8 (0.8)	3	.725

Notes: For descriptive statistics, N = 298. DCW = direct care worker; NH = nursing home.

[a]Each index is constructed by averaging its items' responses. Thus scores on an index fall in the original response range (1 = *strongly disagree* to 5 = *strongly agree*) of its items, with higher scores indicating more of the characteristic.

Table 7.2. Estimated Odds Ratios from Logistic Regression Models Predicting Turnover by Follow-Up Among DCWs

Variable	Model 1	Model 2	Model 3	Model 4	Model 5	Model 6	Model 7
Demographic and Job Characteristics at Baseline							
Non-Hispanic white	1.193	1.163	1.169	1.180	1.225	1.225	1.628
Less than 12th grade	0.785	0.783	0.783	0.766	0.752	0.748	0.818
Some college or more	0.981	0.959	0.955	0.910	0.910	0.890	0.880
At least one child at home	0.814	0.832	0.833	0.828	0.849	0.843	0.869
Difficulty paying bills	1.234	1.182	1.179	1.149	1.236	1.213	1.223
Medical or restorative aide	0.218**	0.208**	0.209**	0.207**	0.214**	0.214**	0.237**
Months employed at NH	0.974***	0.973***	0.973***	0.973***	0.973***	0.973***	0.973***
Perceptions of Work Environment at Baseline							
Adequate DCW staffing	1.017	1.036	1.036	1.073	1.069	1.081	1.179
Treated fairly	1.112	1.153	1.157	1.192	1.176	1.185	1.130
Can trust other DCWs	1.081	1.074	1.077	1.084	1.156	1.154	1.114
Close friend at NH	1.251	1.254	1.255	1.251	1.463	1.436	1.556
Empowerment	0.486*	0.527*	0.530*	0.544	0.557	0.561	0.556
Work-Related Attitudes at Baseline							
Emotional exhaustion		1.245	1.235	1.094	1.213	1.151	1.117
Job satisfaction			0.978	1.141	1.407	1.451	1.443
Intent to quit job at NH				1.440*	—	1.172	1.257
Commitment to NH					0.478**	0.515**	0.562**
Between Baseline and Follow-Up							
Months							1.084*
Teams used within NHs							0.531*
Model χ^2; *df*	95.160; 22***	96.642; 23***	96.651; 24***	100.134; 25***	106.158; 25***	106.691; 26***	94.207; 18***

Notes: N = 298. DCW = direct care worker; NH = nursing home.

Models 1–6 were estimated including facility dummies; however, estimates associated with them are not shown to conserve space.

*$p \le .05$; **$p \le .01$; ***$p \le .001$ (one-tailed tests)

to examine the effect of EWTs on the likelihood of a direct care worker leaving her or his NH, the facility dummies are replaced by the dummy variable indicating whether EWTs were used in the direct care worker's NH between the baseline and follow-up surveys. Also included was a control for the number of months between Time 1 (before teams) and Time 2 (time of follow-up survey). Diagnostic tests revealed no problems with extreme correlations or values among the variables.

Results

Table 7.2 presents the results of the logistic regression models examining how direct care workers' empowerment, EWTs, and work-related attitudes at baseline affected the likelihood of leaving their job by follow-up. Model 1, which includes demographic, job, and work environment characteristics, shows that the odds of leaving decreased with length of service and empowerment and was about 78% lower for direct care workers whose primary tasks were to dispense medications or provide restorative therapies compared with direct care workers with other responsibilities such as those of CNAs.

Models 2 and 3 incorporate the burnout and job satisfaction variables, respectively. Although the effects of these variables on the likelihood of direct care workers' leaving their job are in the expected directions, they lack statistical significance. The effects of the primary responsibility, tenure, and empowerment variables on the odds of leaving remain statistically significant and essentially unchanged.

However, changes do occur with the introduction of the intent to quit and commitment variables in Models 4–6. Although the effects of the primary responsibility and tenure variables on the risk of turnover remain the same, empowerment lacks significance. This pattern suggests that the effects of empowerment on the risk of turnover were mediated by the intent to quit and commitment variables. That is, the effects of a direct care worker's empowerment on turnover occurred through the effects of empowerment on the direct care worker's commitment level and intention to quit. As expected, the odds of leaving the NH at follow-up were about 44% higher with each 1-point increase in baseline intent to quit score (Model 4), and about 49% lower with each 1-point increase in baseline commitment (Model 5). However, when both variables were included in the model simultaneously (Model 6), only commitment retains significance.

Unlike the other models in Table 7.2, Model 7 is estimated excluding the facility dummies. The dummies are replaced by a variable indicating whether a direct care worker's NH used EWTs between the baseline and follow-up surveys and a control for the number of months between the two surveys. This specification allows us to examine whether the EWTs affected the odds of direct care workers no longer working at follow-up, controlling for the effects of other characteristics, including their level of empowerment, at baseline. The results for Model 7 show that the EWTs had such an effect. The odds of leaving were about 47% lower for direct care workers who worked in NHs where EWTs were used than for direct care workers who did not work in such homes. Other factors associated with a lower risk of turnover among direct care workers in Model 7 were having mostly non-CNA responsibilities (e.g., medical or restorative aide), longer tenure, and strong commitment. The only factor associated with a higher risk was months between the baseline and follow-up surveys in the NH.

Discussion

In this study, the effects of direct care worker participation in EWTs were examined in relation to job turnover. Controlling for the effects of the baseline variables, it was found that direct care worker turnover was less likely if EWTs were being used.

These results, together with the results from Chapter 6, indicate that direct care workers who viewed themselves as having a higher level of empowerment tended to be less burned out, more satisfied, less likely to be thinking about quitting, and more committed to the NH. Furthermore, the direct care workers in EWTs were less likely to leave their job by the follow-up or Time 2 survey.

The analyses have some limitations. Because the direct care workers in the sample were employed by 11 volunteer facilities in north Texas, the findings may not apply to direct care workers in NHs in other regions of the country. Additionally, the nature of the intervention and its assessment severely limited the number of NHs included in the study. Thus, although facility dummies were included in our models to control for overall facility-level effects, we are not in a position to reliably evaluate them in greater detail. If the sample had been drawn from a larger number of NHs, we could have identified how specific NH characteristics affect turnover (see Castle & Engberg, 2006).

Furthermore, the measure of turnover includes voluntary as well as involuntary turnover. This study did not distinguish whether a direct care worker left by choice or was fired. Although Castle (2007) argues that in general the calculation of turnover rates should include both voluntary and involuntary turnover, Donoghue and Castle (2006) found that predictors have different associations with these two types of turnover at the facility level. It seems likely that this may also be the case at the individual level. If possible, future prospective studies of individual-level turnover should distinguish between the two types of turnover. Nevertheless, when both are included to represent turnover, the findings show that the odds of a direct care worker leaving the NH were 47% less if the direct care worker worked in an NH where EWTs were being used.

EFFECTS OF EMPOWERMENT ON JOB
PERFORMANCE AND WORK ATTITUDES

Little empirical research has been done on the effects of empowerment on job performance and employee attitudes. This section addresses this gap by using data from the 10 NHs described in Chapter 6 to compare highly empowered direct care workers with those with less empowerment to determine whether they differ on job performance and work attitudes. The perceptions, performance, and attitudes of the nurses with whom the direct care workers worked are also examined. Nurses who viewed themselves as working with highly empowered assistants are compared with those of nurses who viewed themselves as working with less empowered assistants. Furthermore, all of these comparisons are made between direct care workers representing a wide range of empowerment; about one half of the direct care workers and nurses worked in NHs in which EWTs had been implemented, and the other half worked in NHs with more traditional management approaches.

The analyses of EWTs described in Chapter 6 revealed that the EWTs had a variety of positive effects on job performance. However, the teams appeared to have somewhat mixed effects on job attitudes. When assessing the positive effects on attitudes, the analyses indicated that the direct care workers in EWTs often were able to realize their work preferences. In addition, many of the direct care workers appeared to appreciate that the nurses listened to and sometimes implemented their team's suggestions. On the negative side, some direct care workers were worried that the weekly 30-minute team meetings kept them from getting their work done. Other direct care workers had difficulty getting to a meeting when it was scheduled before or after their regular shift, and others expressed frustration when a team member repeatedly brought up an issue or personal problem or when, on occasion, members of nurse management failed to read and respond to the team's notes.

Thus, given these opposing effects of the teams on job attitudes, it is not surprising that the survey data showed no differences between Time 1 and Time 2 for the experimental or comparison NHs with regard to a number of work-related attitudes, including job satisfaction. However, it seems premature to conclude that direct care worker empowerment per se has a neutral effect on the work-related attitudes of direct care workers and nurses in NHs. Further examination is needed. Thus, using data from direct care workers representing a wide range of empowerment, this section examines whether the direct care workers who felt high levels of empowerment perceived their job performance and attitudes differently than those who experienced a moderate or low level of empowerment. Additionally, the analyses examined whether the nurses working with highly empowered direct care workers differed in their perceptions from nurses working with less empowered direct care workers.

Methods

Data for this analysis come from the Time 2 self-administered questionnaires of direct care workers and nurses in the study conducted by Yeatts and Cready, described in Chapter 6. At Time 2 half of the direct care workers had been working in EWTs for roughly 17–18 months and so were likely to have experienced high levels of empowerment. Chapter 6 describes in detail the procedures used to collect these data.

In order to examine differences between high, medium, and low direct care worker empowerment, direct care workers with the highest scores on empowerment were placed in one group, those with the lowest in a second, and the remainder in a third, middle group. The highest-empowerment group was compared with each of the other groups with regard to demographic characteristics, perceived job performance, work attitudes, self-reported absenteeism, and intent to quit. All direct care worker variables except absenteeism were indices and were constructed in the same manner as the empowerment indices (described in Chapter 6), with higher scores indicating more of the characteristic. Cronbach's alphas typically were over .70, with the lowest being .55 (for the "direct care worker time for care" index).

Similar procedures were used to examine differences between high, medium, and low direct care worker empowerment from the perspective of the nurses. Using the nurse index of direct care worker empowerment, we placed nurses into three groups based on how empowered they perceived the direct care workers they worked with to be, and nurses in the highest group were compared with each of the other groups. Like the direct care workers, the nurses were compared on their perceptions of direct care worker job performance in their NH. The nurses were also compared on their perceptions of their own job performance, satisfaction, absenteeism, and intent to quit. Like the direct care worker variables, all nurse variables except absenteeism were indices and were constructed in the same manner as the empowerment indices. Cronbach's alpha was over .70 for each of the nurse indices except one (i.e., $\alpha = .66$ for the "direct care worker time for care" index).

For almost all comparisons between the highest-empowerment direct care worker group and each of the other two groups, independent t tests were used to evaluate statistical significance. The only exceptions were the comparisons on direct care worker gender and direct care worker race or ethnicity. Chi-square tests were used for these comparisons.

Results

The top panel of Table 7.3 presents the sample sizes and mean scores on the indices measuring direct care worker perceptions of their empowerment (i.e., global empowerment and each of its dimensions of autonomy, competence, and impact or meaningfulness) for the three direct care worker empowerment groups (i.e., low, medium, and high). As expected, with mean scores from 3.9 to 4.3 on the indices, direct care workers in the high-empowerment group tended to agree that they were empowered. Direct care workers in the medium-empowerment group tended to be somewhat uncertain that they were empowered. And direct care workers in the low-empowerment group tended to be more uncertain or to disagree that they were empowered.

An examination of the demographic characteristics in the bottom panel of Table 7.3 reveals no differences between the three direct care worker empowerment groups with regard to sex, race or ethnicity, education, and difficulty paying bills ($p > .05$). However, there were significant differences with regard to age and tenure ($p < .05$). Highly empowered direct care workers tended to be somewhat older and have longer tenure at the NH than less empowered direct care workers.

A comparison of the three groups of direct care workers with regard to job performance finds many differences (Table 7.4, top panel), with highly empowered

Table 7.3.   DCW Levels of Empowerment and Demographic Characteristics

Variable	DCW Perceptions of DCW Empowerment		
	Low Mean	Medium Mean	High Mean
DCW Perceptions of DCW Empowerment			
Global empowerment	2.7	3.5	4.1
Autonomy in doing work	2.7	3.2	3.9
Competence in doing work	3.0	3.7	4.3
Impact or meaningfulness of work	2.6	3.5	4.2
Number of cases	100	140	58
Demographic Characteristics of DCWs			
Percentage female	91.9	88.6	86.2
Percentage non-Anglo	66.7	52.2	62.1
Mean education (in years completed)	12.0	12.1	11.9
Mean difficulty paying bills	3.6	3.4	3.2
Mean age (in years)	36.8++	35.3**	43.2
Mean number of months at NH	38.2	37.0*	59.3
Number of cases	100	140	58

Notes: DCW = direct care worker; NH = nursing home.

The empowerment indices and difficulty paying bills range from 1 to 5; the larger the mean, the more of the characteristic. The number of cases varies somewhat from variable to variable because of missing values.

+Significant difference between high and low empowerment at the .05 level using a two-tailed t test.

++Significant difference between high and low empowerment at the .01 level using a two-tailed t test.

*Significant difference between high and medium empowerment at the .05 level using a two-tailed t test.

**Significant difference between high and medium empowerment at the .01 level using a two-tailed t test.

direct care workers scoring significantly higher on all three of the performance measures than those with less empowerment ($p < .05$). Highly empowered direct care workers were more likely to agree that they have effective work procedures, enough time to feed, turn, and assist residents, and support for each other than lesser empowered direct care workers.

A similar pattern was observed among the nurses. As the bottom panel of Table 7.4 shows, the nurses' assessments of direct care worker job performance tended to differ depending on how empowered they perceived the direct care workers in their NH to be. Nurses who perceived the direct care workers in their NH to be highly empowered (column 3, the high-empowerment group) tended to rate the direct care workers higher on five different aspects of their performance than nurses who perceived the direct care workers in their NH to have low empowerment ($p < .05$). Nurse ratings were higher on average for highly empowered direct care workers regarding their staffing levels and time available to provide resident care. Nurses also tended to rate these direct care workers slightly higher on the effectiveness of their work procedures, their coordination with other direct care workers, and their cooperation with other nursing staff.

Nurses were asked about their own job performance as well. Specifically, they were asked to give their opinions about having enough time to complete their paperwork. As the bottom panel of Table 7.4 shows, nurses who viewed themselves as working with direct care workers with the lowest levels of empowerment tended to disagree (2.4) that there was enough time for nurses to complete their paper-work. Nurses who viewed themselves as working with highly empowered direct care workers were less certain (3.0) about the lack of time for this task. However, this difference is not statistically significant ($p > .05$). Thus, according to the nurses, working with highly empowered direct care workers did not tend to free up more of nurses' time for getting their paperwork done.

Table 7.5 presents job attitudes, absenteeism, and intent to quit among direct care workers and nurses by levels of direct care worker empowerment. As predicted, direct care worker empowerment was strongly associated with both direct care workers' and nurses' attitudes toward their job. It had the biggest impacts on some of the attitudes of the direct care workers (Table 7.5, top panel). Direct care workers with high empowerment scored higher than others on self-esteem, satisfaction with their job and schedule, and commitment to the NH, and lower on burnout ($p < .05$). Highly empowered direct care workers were also less likely to be thinking of leaving their job ($p < .05$), suggesting lower turnover among this group.

Results were similar for the nurses. Nurses who viewed the direct care workers in their NH as highly empowered appeared to be the happiest. As the bottom panel of Table 7.5 shows, these nurses tended to score higher on job satisfaction

Table 7.4. Levels of DCW Empowerment and Job Performance

Characteristic	DCW Perceptions of DCW Empowerment		
	Low Mean	Medium Mean	High Mean
DCW Perceptions of DCW Job Performance			
DCWs have effective work procedures	3.4++	3.7**	4.2
DCWs have enough time to provide care	3.4++	3.7	3.9
DCWs support each other	3.3++	3.7**	4.1
Number of cases	100	140	58

Characteristic	Nurse Perceptions of DCW Empowerment		
	Low Mean	Medium Mean	High Mean
Nurse Perceptions of DCW Job Performance			
DCWs have effective work procedures	3.6++	3.9**	4.3
DCWs work well together	3.3++	3.7**	4.2
Adequate DCW staffing to do a good job	2.7++	3.3**	4.1
DCWs have enough time to provide care	2.9++	3.4**	4.0
DCWs cooperate with nurses	3.7++	4.1**	4.5
Nurse Perceptions of Nurse Job Performance			
Nurses have enough time to complete paperwork	2.4	2.9	3.0
Number of cases	32	72	32

Notes: DCW = direct care worker.

The indices used to measure the job performance characteristics range from 1 (*strongly disagree*) to 5 (*strongly agree*). The larger the mean is, the more of the characteristic. The number of cases varies slightly from characteristic to characteristic because of missing values.

+Significant difference between high and low empowerment at the .05 level using a two-tailed *t* test.

++Significant difference between high and low empowerment at the .01 level using a two-tailed *t* test.

*Significant difference between high and medium empowerment at the .05 level using a two-tailed *t* test.

**Significant difference between high and medium empowerment at the .01 level using a two-tailed *t* test.

than nurses working with medium- or low-empowerment direct care workers ($p <$ .05). In addition, the nurses in the high-empowerment direct care worker group were the least likely to be thinking of leaving their job ($p < .05$).

The only variable showing no significant difference between the three empowerment groups was self-reported absenteeism ($p > .05$). Regardless of their perceptions of the levels of direct care worker empowerment in their NH, when asked how often they missed work for reasons other than vacation both direct care workers and nurses alike tended to respond "about 1 day every 2 months or more." However, it is important to note that of all the survey questions used in this analysis, this question was the one with the lowest response rate among direct care workers. Moreover, the response rate for this question was lowest among the least-empowered direct care workers and highest among those most empowered. Thus it is possible that lower absenteeism was associated with higher levels of direct care worker empowerment, at least among the direct care workers, but was obscured by these differing response rates.

Table 7.5. Levels of DCW Empowerment and Job Attitudes, Absenteeism, and Intention to Quit

Characteristic	DCW Perceptions of DCW Empowerment		
	Low Mean	Medium Mean	High Mean
DCW Attitudes, Absenteeism, and Intention to Quit			
Self-esteem	4.0++	4.1**	4.5
Experiencing burnout on the job	2.4++	2.2**	1.7
Emotional exhaustion	2.8++	2.5**	1.9
Depersonalization	2.0++	1.9**	1.5
Generally satisfied with job	3.5++	3.8**	4.6
Satisfied with schedule	3.0+	3.2	3.6
Committed to job	3.5++	3.8**	4.5
Self-reported absenteeism	1.5	1.3	1.4
Planning to quit job	2.7++	2.3**	1.7
Number of cases	100	140	58

Characteristic	Nurse Perceptions of DCW Empowerment		
	Low Mean	Medium Mean	High Mean
Nurse Satisfaction, Absenteeism, and Intention to Quit			
Generally satisfied with job	3.6++	4.0**	4.4
Self-reported absenteeism	1.1	1.1	1.1
Planning to quit job	2.4++	1.9	1.8
Number of cases	32	72	32

Notes: DCW = direct care worker.

The indices used to measure job attitudes and intention to quit range from 1 (*strongly disagree*) to 5 (*strongly agree*). Absenteeism ranges from 1 (*about 1 day/2 months or more*) to 5 (*about 1 day/week*). The larger the mean is, the more of the characteristic. The number of cases varies somewhat from characteristic to characteristic because of missing values.

+Significant difference between high and low empowerment at the .05 level using a two-tailed *t* test.

++Significant difference between high and low empowerment at the .01 level using a two-tailed *t* test.

*Significant difference between high and medium empowerment at the .05 level using a two-tailed *t* test.

**Significant difference between high and medium empowerment at the .01 level using a two-tailed *t* test.

Discussion

The purpose of this analysis was to examine the effects of direct care worker empowerment among a sample of direct care workers representing a wide range of empowerment. Based on the survey responses of both direct care workers and nurses from five NHs where EWTs had been implemented and five NHs with more traditional management approaches, the results of the analysis indicated that direct care worker empowerment had a variety of effects. According to both direct care workers and nurses, highly empowered direct care workers tended to perform their jobs better than other direct care workers. Compared with less empowered direct care workers, highly empowered direct care workers were perceived to have effective work procedures, to have enough time and staff to provide care, to support and work well with other direct care workers, and to cooperate with the nurses. However, these higher levels of direct care worker performance did not seem to increase the amount of time available for the nurses to complete their paperwork.

Collectively, both highly empowered direct care workers and the nurses who worked with them also seemed to be happier on the job. Highly empowered direct care workers reported higher self-esteem, less burnout, more satisfaction, and more commitment. The nurses who worked with such direct care workers also reported more satisfaction. And both were less likely to be thinking about leaving their jobs.

Although the job performance findings of this analysis were consistent with the results of the pretest and posttest of EWTs described in Chapter 6, the job attitude findings are not. The analyses show that although feelings of empowerment are associated with positive job attitudes, EWTs are not necessarily. EWTs were found to sometimes produce negative feelings if they were not implemented or managed well. For example, this occurred when direct care workers were asked to attend meetings before or after their shift or when nurse management neglected to respond to the direct care worker notes from their weekly team meetings.

IMPLICATIONS FOR PRACTICE

It is clear from the analyses that direct care worker empowerment is associated with positive work-related attitudes among direct care workers and nurses. These findings, together with those in Chapter 6, suggest that direct care worker empowerment, as a management approach, can be used to increase the morale and performance of direct care workers and nurses, lower staff intent to quit their jobs, and improve the quality of NH residents' care and lives. However, as noted earlier, the effectiveness of an employee empowerment strategy such as EWTs depends largely on how well it is implemented. Like other empowering strategies, EWTs are most effective when they have the support of management (Robinson & Rosher, 2006; Yeatts & Cready, 2007). One challenge for members of nurse management who are seeking to improve their NHs' work and care environment by implementing EWTs is finding the time to ask for and listen to direct care worker suggestions on how to modify the work and to provide consistent feedback. Another challenge is getting direct care workers involved in the decision-making process in situations that warrant immediate attention, such as when a complaint must be addressed quickly. Still other challenges include giving the direct care workers time to learn how to work together in a team meeting, allowing for the possibility that they will sometimes make mistakes, and making sure that their direct care responsibilities are covered while they attend their team's weekly scheduled meeting.

Thus NHs and other long-term care providers, such as assisted living facilities and home care communities, that are interested in empowering their workers face some significant challenges. Fortunately, they can learn from the successes and problems experienced by the few who have pioneered various empowerment strategies, including EWTs in NHs. With the help of lessons learned from the new culture change initiatives, and with commitment, effort, and attention, NHs and other long-term care providers can reap the benefits associated with employee empowerment strategies such as EWTs. The last section of this book provides important implementation strategies and tools for initiating EWTs.

CHAPTER 8

Knowledge as Empowerment
Improving Direct Care Workers' Education and Training

Linda S. Noelker, Farida K. Ejaz, and Heather L. Menne

Few studies have examined the factors that enhance or inhibit the empowerment of direct care workers in long-term care. This chapter begins with an introduction to the relationships between education, training, and empowerment. It then provides findings from a survey of 432 direct care workers in 22 nursing homes (NHs) in northern Ohio. The survey focused on the amount of education and training being provided to direct care workers and on their perceptions and recommendations regarding the types of education and training needed and ways to improve existing job orientation and continuing education programs. The findings point to ways of enhancing direct care worker empowerment, increasing their job satisfaction, and ultimately improving resident care.

According to Kanter's (1993) theory of worker empowerment, two essential components of empowerment are *access to information necessary to do the job* and the *opportunity to learn and grow*. When organizations are structured (or restructured) in ways that optimize these components, the theory posits that employees will have better work attitudes and that organizational effectiveness will increase. Two other essential components for worker empowerment are *providing the resources needed for the job* (e.g., equipment, supplies) and *workplace support*. Research studies testing this theory in health care environments, primarily hospitals, have observed the following outcomes for nursing staff as a consequence of empowerment: greater trust in management (Laschinger, Finegan, Shamian, & Casier, 2000), more commitment to the job (Baguey, 1999), greater accountability for their work (Laschinger, Wong, McMahon, & Kaufmann, 1999), less job-related strain (Laschinger, Finegan, Shamian, & Wills, 2001; Laschinger & Havens, 1996), and higher levels of job satisfaction (Whyte, 1995).

Empowerment theory also posits that it is management's responsibility to ensure that the work environment is designed to promote employee empowerment. Our contention is that when NHs provide high-quality training and educational opportunities for direct care workers that lead to job advancement, their access to information and opportunities to learn and grow are enhanced, resulting in higher levels of empowerment. These opportunities typically occur during the direct care workers' entry-level training and in job orientation and continuing education programs. However, other innovative opportunities can be offered through career ladder programs that move workers into higher-level occupations such as professional nursing and career lattice programs that include advancement within the direct care worker's role, such as the completion of specialty certificate programs (e.g., dementia care specialist or medication aide) (Maier, 2002; McDonald, 1991–1992; Nakhnikian, Wilner, & Hurd, 2002; Remsburg, Armacost, & Bennett, 1999; Stone & Wiener, 2001). One way NHs can offer advancement opportunities into professional nursing is by partnering with community colleges and local universities to bring licensed vocational and registered nursing programs into the workplace.

In the absence of high-quality education and training programs, direct care workers will lack important skills for providing high-quality care for residents and the competence and confidence needed for the job. They also will be more likely to experience lower levels of job satisfaction and commitment (Stone & Wiener, 2001; Wilner & Wyatt, 1998). Furthermore, education and training programs must be responsive to the perceived needs and recommendations of experienced direct care workers who know what skills are needed for the job. In fact, the active involvement of direct care workers in the development and delivery of training programs can be self-empowering, giving them a voice in decision making and adding an important new dimension to their work role.

The pressing need for expanded and enhanced education and training programs for direct care workers in NHs is clearly evident. The Institute of Medicine's (2001, p. 251) report on the quality of NHs states that the long-term care workforce does not have the skills necessary to care for an increasingly frail and medically complex population. Davis's (1991) review of 20 years of research on NH quality similarly concludes that strategies to develop the skills and competencies of the staff should be a prominent focus of future research investigations. The research reported in this chapter addressed this need and examined direct care workers' perceptions of the adequacy and utility of their entry-level training, job orientation, and continuing education; their recommendations for improving the content, format, and delivery of education and training programs; and the effect of these perceptions on job outcomes.

EXAMINING THE TRAINING
NEEDS OF DIRECT CARE WORKERS

A series of studies was conducted by the Margaret Blenkner Research Institute to survey direct care workers about their perceptions of the skills, competencies, and methods of instruction most valuable for helping them succeed in their job. Although these studies were grounded in a stress and social support conceptual model (Ejaz, Noelker, Menne, & Bagakas, 2008; Noelker, Ejaz, Menne, & Jones, 2006) and not an empowerment model, several of its components are closely related to empowerment concepts. For example, workplace support is a key component in both models, and the research studies examined both negative and positive support from peers, other staff, and residents. As noted previously, opportunities to learn and gain access to information, which are central components of the empowerment model, are captured in the stress and support model in two ways. First, best practices in management include the facility's provision of career ladders for direct care workers (opportunities to learn and grow) and enhanced job orientation, mentorship, and continuing education programs that reflect access to information needed to do the job effectively. This research sought to understand direct care workers' perceptions of their initial and continuing education, mentorship, job orientation, and facility practices regarding job advancement, information seen as affecting adequate access to information and opportunities to grow. The stress and support model's other major components include demographic characteristics of the workers such as age and gender, characteristics of the facilities in which they are employed (e.g., for-profit or nonprofit), their personal and job-related stressors, management practices such as the provision of career ladders, and the study's outcome, job satisfaction.

A series of three research surveys guided by the stress and social support model involved 338 direct care workers from 22 nursing facilities in northeast Ohio. Findings from these surveys lent support to the especially powerful effect of direct care workers' personal stressors (e.g., poorer emotional health, financial worries, and concerns about family members while at work) on job satisfaction and satisfaction with supervision (Noelker & Ejaz, 2001; Noelker et al., 2006). Direct care workers with more depressive symptoms, worries about paying bills and managing debt, and concerns about family members left alone while they work have lower levels of job satisfaction and satisfaction with supervision.

Job-related stressors also have a negative but less powerful impact on these outcomes; the job-related stressors included reports of frequent changes made to work schedules (e.g., being asked to come in early or stay over shift) and direct care workers' perceptions that their entry-level training for the job was inadequate. Positive support in the workplace was shown to reduce the negative effects of job-related stressors on the satisfaction outcome, although negative support had no effect. Positive support referred to positive feelings (e.g., respect, affection) that direct care workers derived from interaction with residents and other direct care workers.

Findings from these earlier surveys provide evidence that if NHs are to empower direct care workers to do their jobs effectively, they need to build in support systems that address personal and job-related stress and training needs. Furthermore, the findings suggest that two components of the empowerment model, having the information needed for the job and workplace support, are likely to increase direct care workers' job satisfaction and satisfaction with supervision.

Whereas the strengths of these earlier surveys were their use of the stress and support conceptual model and a large sample of respondents from multiple study sites, the NHs studied were not randomly selected, so the generalizability of the findings is limited. Moreover, these surveys did not attend to the important influence of organizational factors such as career ladders and low turnover rates on direct care workers' job outcomes. Lastly, the prior surveys did not fully explore direct care workers' perceptions about their education and training for the job and recommendations to improve their training, all of which are features of the current Better Education = Better Care survey, funded under the Better Jobs Better Care Initiative (Ejaz & Noelker, 2006).

STUDY DESIGN OF THE BETTER
EDUCATION = BETTER CARE PROJECT

This study involved a cross-sectional survey of direct care workers employed in NHs, assisted living facilities, and home health agencies in a five-county area of northeast Ohio. Using a proportionate random sampling strategy and information from a preliminary survey of the 319 responding organizations, 25 NHs, 13 assisted living facilities, and 8 home health care agencies were selected to participate in the study. This yielded the 46 sites needed for statistical analysis. As the sampling progressed, three additional sites had to be added to the sample in order to boost the number of direct care workers needed for the analysis, resulting in a total of 49 sites. Comparisons were made of the participating and nonparticipating sites, and no differences were found on key indicators such as profit status and the number of direct care workers employed.

An attempt also was made to use proportionate random sampling of direct care workers at the sites, based on the number each site employed; however, budgetary and time constraints prevented the study from reaching the target sample goal of 920 direct care workers (see Ejaz et al., 2008, for details). The final sample included 432 direct care workers from 27 NHs, 106 resident assistants from 14 assisted living facilities, and 106 home health workers from 8 home care agencies. When providing information about education and training, this report focuses exclusively on data from the 432 direct care workers at the 27 NHs that made up the overwhelming majority of the study sample.

Survey data from the 432 direct care workers were collected using either in-person or telephone interviews that lasted an average of 50 minutes. Respondents were paid for completing an interview, and some sites allowed the interviews to be conducted on site during work time, which increased the participation rate. Informed consent procedures approved by the Benjamin Rose Institute's institutional review board were followed carefully.

In addition to the direct care worker interviews, data were also collected from a project site liaison at each organization. This organizational information typically was supplied by a management staff member, who completed a mailed survey on organizational characteristics and management practices. Site liaisons at all 27 NHs completed the survey, which yielded important information about the NHs' characteristics such as staffing structure, ratio of professional licensed nurses to direct care workers, reimbursement sources, and management practices such as the number and types of recruitment and retention strategies, benefit packages, and career ladders for direct care workers.

BACKGROUND CHARACTERISTICS
OF THE DIRECT CARE WORKERS

As Table 8.1 shows, the direct care workers in this sample were overwhelmingly women (93.5%), and the majority (61.3%) were minority, mostly African American workers. Their average age was approximately 37 years, with a range from 19 to 67 years, and about one third were married. Most of the direct care workers (92.1%) had at least a high school diploma, and a number had taken college courses. Most (82.2%) worked full time, and workers from all three shifts were well represented in the sample. Almost half worked first shift, and about a quarter each worked second and third shift. On average, the direct care workers had been employed in the facility for almost 5 years, although their tenure ranged from 1 month to more than 30 years. In terms of their job tenure as direct care workers, regardless of where they were employed, the average length of time was almost 10 years.

DIRECT CARE WORKERS' PERCEPTIONS OF THEIR EDUCATION AND TRAINING

Entry-Level Training

The direct care workers were asked a series of questions about their entry-level or initial training, including its content, design, format, and adequacy. Ninety-two percent of the direct care workers received initial training after the requirements of the 1987 Omnibus Budget Reconciliation Act (OBRA) went into effect. The OBRA requirements mandate a minimum of 75 hours initial training, 12 hours annually of continuing education, and competency testing within 4 months of employment (Institute of Medicine, 2001, p. 197). The State of Ohio has not raised the initial training minimum requirement beyond 75 hours, it tests but does

Table 8.1. Characteristics of Direct Care Workers (*n* = 432)

Variables	Actual Score Range	Mean (*SD*) or %
Age	19–67	37.62 (12.20)
Gender (1 = female)	0–1	93.5%
Marital status (1 = married)	0–1	34.1%
Race or ethnicity (1 = minority)	0–1	61.3%
Education level		
Less than high school diploma		7.8%
High school diploma or GED		45.8%
Some college courses		42.4%
College graduate or higher		4.0%
Work status (1 = full time)	0–1	82.2%
Length of time working in facility or agency (months)	1–384	56.59 (70.69)
Length of time as direct care worker in any setting (months)	1–480	115.28 (99.19)
Shift		
First		49.3%
Second		24.5%
Third		26.2%

not certify direct care workers, and it has not mandated additional training components such as communication skills and training in dementia care, as other states have.

Only 55% of the direct care workers reported that their entry-level training prepared them well for the job of caring for residents in an NH. Most were satisfied with the amount of classroom time included in the training (93%), and a slightly smaller portion (83%) was satisfied with the time spent doing hands-on care. The direct care workers pointed out several key work skills that were not covered in the entry-level training. One skill, cited by one third of the respondents, was instruction in how to organize their tasks efficiently so that all the work can be completed on time. In view of the intensive demands of resident care and the fact that most units do not have enough direct care staff, it is not surprising many experienced direct care workers would mention this as an important skill that should be integral to entry-level training. As some of the respondents noted,

"Teach better organization of time that mirrors what the real work situation will be like."

"Cover how to handle the work load when short-staffed."

"They need to get the STNAs [State-Tested Nursing Assistants] on the floor sooner in their training so that they know what the work is about. Explain to trainees that this is difficult and stressful work."

Skill at organizing tasks encompasses the ability to consider all tasks that need to be accomplished on a shift, prioritize them, and plan their execution in a manner that is time efficient. Moreover, this process is likely to have to be repeated throughout the shift as unexpected events happen (e.g., a resident is sent to the hospital) or the staffing situation changes (e.g., call-offs and no-shows occur). This skill entails both foresight and flexibility, and when direct care workers lack the ability to organize their work efficiently, the work is either not done or not done well. The latter is well documented by Foner (1994) in her observational study of direct care workers and how they carry out their work, and by others (Bowers & Becker, 1992). When the press of work demands becomes too great, direct care workers often look for shortcuts; for example, unfinished work gets hidden and left for the next shift.

A second essential job skill not covered in entry-level training for 27% of the direct care workers was teamwork. In order to work more efficiently, direct care workers on the same unit or floor can benefit from jointly planning and executing their tasks. However, teamwork entails a complex set of skills, which include an understanding of different communication styles, the ability to negotiate and compromise, and a willingness to take initiative. Although some trainers may regard these as "soft skills" in comparison to the technical skills of taking vital signs or lifting and transferring a resident, interpersonal skills are at the heart of building positive relationships with residents and peers and at the heart of caregiving. When these skills are excluded from entry-level training programs or their value is minimized, the wrong message is sent about their importance, leaving trainees ill equipped for the highly interactive nature of their work with staff and residents. As three of the respondents advised,

> "Stress the importance of working as a team for safety's sake for residents and the STNAs."

> "More teamwork because that is really needed in that field. Everyone needs to be unified. Everything would be so much easier. Everyone is out to help only themselves and their residents."

> "Have the same preceptor to work with for the initial training days, about 3 to 4 days. Right now there is a different preceptor for each of those 3 days. Teamwork is something you don't see. It's important."

A third essential job skill that was not covered in entry-level training for 23% of the respondents was dealing with residents who act out or are abusive. Because the percentage of NH residents admitted with Alzheimer's disease or other form of dementia is estimated at 48% to 55% (Magaziner et al., 2000), with some estimates as high as 74% (Garrard et al., 1993), newly trained direct care workers are very likely to be involved in the care of residents who present some level of behavioral challenge.

Although not all residents have challenging behavior, a direct care worker who is untrained in their care can evoke a catastrophic reaction if she or he attempts to bathe or give another type of personal care to a resident who is resistive or apprehensive (Brunk, 1997; Kovach & Meyer-Arnold, 1996; Talerico & Evans, 2000). Residents may respond by hitting, grabbing, scratching, biting, or spitting at the direct care worker, and both parties may be injured as a result. Residents' family members can further complicate the situation by accusing the direct care worker of deliberately injuring the resident because they are unaware of how the resident behaves when they are not there. It is for these reasons that safer approaches to bathing NH residents with dementia have been developed and evaluated with direct care workers, showing promise for reducing resident resistance and aggression (Barrick, Rader, Hoeffer, & Sloane, 2000; Hoeffer et al., 2006). As respondents in our study commented,

> "I never knew how hard it is to care for residents on the behavioral unit. I wasn't prepared for what goes on here with these residents."

> "Teach how to deal with combative residents, the ones with mental health conditions, with drug and alcohol problems."

> "Families need to be educated as to what the resident's behaviors are when the family is there and when the family is not there. Families need to understand what the STNA faces."

> "More honesty [is needed] in the classroom about what actually goes on in a nursing home with residents. Some may act out, are abusive, and combative. The nurses know about that stuff but we don't know about it. We need to know their behavior problems."

Job Orientation Programs

The importance of a thorough job orientation program cannot be emphasized enough; however, additional considerations are in order. For example, one of the more noteworthy reports from a direct care worker about her job orientation was how impressed she had been initially by the orientation program at her facility, which ran for 2 weeks with the option of an extension if she felt it were necessary. After 2 weeks of orientation, she was confident she knew the residents and staff on her unit, where supplies and equipment were kept, and what the procedures were for shift changes, breaks, and reporting on residents' status. She was looking forward to beginning her first week on the unit as a regular direct care worker, but when she reported for work the next Monday, she found she had been assigned to a different unit where she knew no one and nothing about the unit. She vividly recalled how frightened she was. It may be for reasons such as this that only 49% of the direct care workers in the sample reported that their job orientation program was "very helpful," although 95% had participated in an orientation program at the facility where they were employed.

The importance of including a mentoring program in job orientation, in which an experienced direct care worker is available as an instructor, coach, and counselor, is receiving increasing attention (Noble, 2004; Paraprofessional Health Care Institute, 2003). Among respondents in this study, 81% said their facilities had a mentoring program for new direct care workers. However, they were able to observe some problems with the orientation and mentoring programs that made them less effective, as the following comments indicate:

> "They should work with more than one mentor and get to know all the residents or at least the group they will be assigned to."

> "The trainer should be able to devote more time to teaching the trainee. For example, the trainer should have a lighter resident load while training someone so that they can show the new trainee the right way to do things."

> "For training, they need to let the new NA [Nursing Assistant] get hands-on experience while being observed rather than just have them follow around the other NA to see what they are doing."

Continuing Education Programs

Continuing education sessions have the potential to expand direct care workers' skill sets and knowledge base, thus affording them access to new information and developmental opportunities that can lead to worker empowerment. However, as noted earlier, only 12 hours annually of continuing education is mandated under OBRA 1987, and much of the required content must be repeated, such as fire safety, residents' rights, and universal precautions. Important topic areas not covered in entry-level training seem logical to include in continuing education sessions, such as the organization of the work, teamwork, and dementia care. However, as this research uncovered, there are other obstacles to effective continuing education apart from the limited hours and required content.

Only 5% of the direct care workers said they had not received continuing education at the NH in which they worked because they were too new to the job. Of the 95% who participated in continuing education sessions, almost half (45%) did not find the sessions very useful. More than half (56%) reported that a lack of coverage on the floor or unit was a major barrier to attending or benefiting from the continuing education sessions. As the following comments indicate, the respondents had a number of problems with the delivery of in-service sessions in the NH:

"In-services should be scheduled into work time with coverage taken care of so that we can go."

"In-services are held mostly on day shift so it's hard to attend."

"I recommend more communication between nursing assistants and the nurses. There is none. Some nurses straight out of school do not have management skills—they're power hungry. They don't talk right to nursing assistants. Some of them, not all of them."

Other important in-service topics were noted that the direct care workers thought should be covered but were not, and a number of these involved improving interpersonal and organizational skills. Specifically, 57% of the direct care workers said that dealing with other direct care workers who were difficult to work with was not covered during their in-service sessions. The two other topics were how to work well with a supervisor (50%) and how to better organize work tasks (43%), the latter of which was also endorsed for inclusion in entry-level training. There also were three technical skill areas that were widely reported as not included in continuing education sessions: taking vital signs properly (50%), giving CPR (44%), and caring for residents with mental illness (36%).

DIRECT CARE WORKERS' RECOMMENDATIONS TO IMPROVE EDUCATION AND TRAINING

As Table 8.2 shows, the direct care workers in this research had a variety of recommendations for improving entry-level training, job orientation, and continuing education programs. Their most ringing endorsement was to expand the length of all three. It is eminently clear that the minimum of 75 hours for entry-level training is inadequate, and experts have issued calls to mandate a minimum of 150 hours (Harrington, Kovner, et al., 2000). Some states, such as California, have already raised the minimum hour requirement to 150, and some have mandated specific content areas such as communication skills and dementia care (Institute of Medicine, 2001, p. 197). An argument has also been made to increase the mandatory continuing education hours and to have a registered nurse educator on site 24 hours a day to improve on-the-job training for direct care workers (Institute of Medicine, 2001, p. 197).

The length of job orientation programs should be governed by the particular needs of the new employee, and the program should be linked with mentorship opportunities for high-performing NAs. Because the skill sets, work experience, and maturity of newly hired direct care workers and the quality of their entry-level training will vary, each one should be evaluated routinely throughout the orientation period to determine how long the program should last. Additionally, the new hire should have a voice in how much orientation time is needed.

In addition to raising the 12-hour annual requirement for continuing education, the direct care workers in this study recommended that in-service sessions should be shorter (e.g., 15 to 30 minutes), more frequent, and repeated on all shifts. This approach would require less time off the unit and away from the residents in their care.

The content of education and training programs should focus more on how to organize the work so that it is completed in a timely manner while managing crises on the unit or working short staffed. Organization and time management skills are essential for the direct care workforce, and these skills tie to teamwork so that each direct care worker is prepared to pitch in when something needs to be done and coworkers are occupied with an unexpected demand. Teamwork also is a key component of empowered work teams, helping workers coordinate their activities and shift responsibilities as needed. It also requires workers to become problem solvers rather than simply problem identifiers, relying on the professional

Table 8.2.   Direct Care Workers' Recommendations to Improve Education and Training

Recommendations	Entry-Level Training	Job Orientation	Continuing Education
Length and frequency	Longer.	Longer.	More frequent sessions. Shorter sessions. Offer on each shift and all days of the week.
Content	Resident interactions (difficult residents, communication, respect, teamwork). Dementia care. Help with lifting and transferring. Taking vital signs.	Resident interactions (difficult residents, communication, respect, teamwork).	Resident interactions (difficult residents, communication, respect, teamwork). Mental illness and dementia. Taking vital signs. CPR.
Design, format, and delivery	More hands-on and clinical time. More one-on-one instruction.	Experienced mentor for one-on-one training. Conduct on all units where new employee will work. Hands-on training, training on the floor.	Offer on site. Interactive training (e.g., group, hands-on, role playing). Use print materials. Use computers. Ensure unit coverage. Obtain worker input on content and design. Videotape sessions.

nursing staff to come up with solutions. In order to do this effectively, however, each team member has to be an active participant, and often they are neither willing nor able. This appears to lie at the root of requests for more in-service training that deals with difficult coworkers and training that develops better working relationships with supervisors.

As Table 8.2 indicates, the content areas for training and education programs include both technical skills and interpersonal and organizational skills. Currently, there is an imbalance in the content of entry-level and continuing education programs, with a far heavier emphasis on technical skills. The direct care workers surveyed here were consistent in their requests for more training in technical areas such as dementia care and dealing with other types of mental health disorders, taking vital signs properly, and administering CPR. However, they placed equal emphasis on communication, teamwork, and other interpersonal skills essential for the highly interactive environment of the NH.

In terms of the design and delivery of education and training programs, a portion of the direct care workers requested to be personally involved in planning the content and how it is delivered. Each session and program should be followed by a debriefing period in which the participants critique the session and offer recommendations for improvement. This approach embodies teamwork and places equal responsibility on the direct care workers and the trainer for working to maximize the utility and benefits of the session. The inclusion of high-performing direct care workers as trainers for entry-level and continuing education was also widely endorsed by the respondents in this study. Yet when they are serving as trainers or mentors it was recommended that their work responsibilities be lightened and that they be compensated with a higher rate of pay or a bonus for undertaking the task.

For job orientation and mentorship programs, the direct care workers highly recommended training new hires on all units to which they will be assigned in order to familiarize them with the residents and other employees and how the unit is structured and operates. This seems transparently obvious, but findings from this study show that it was not uncommon to place a new hire on a unit where someone is available to train, without regard for where the new hire would eventually be assigned. The exigencies of NH operations often thwart efforts to engage in good management practices, and so continuing education sessions or in-services are offered without always taking into account the work load on the units that day. Additionally, direct care workers may be asked to sacrifice breaks or mealtimes to attend sessions, which many see as an unwelcome imposition.

Recommendations were made to plan in-services around unit coverage, to offer them on site, to design them so that they foster interaction between direct care workers, and to take a multimedia approach (e.g., use print materials to read when convenient, use computer training programs, videotape sessions to show on different shifts). As the findings indicate, direct care workers have clear and cogent opinions about their education and training and thoughtful recommendations about how to improve them when they are asked. Provider organizations can capitalize on the wisdom and experience of direct care workers by ensuring that they are actively involved in planning the content, design, delivery, and evaluation of these programs.

IMPACT OF INADEQUATE EDUCATION AND TRAINING ON DIRECT CARE WORKER JOB SATISFACTION

Findings from this research clearly underscore the perceived inadequacies in entry-level training, job orientation, and continuing education programs, which bodes poorly for worker empowerment and for important job outcomes such as job satisfaction. In fact, data analysis focused on job-related stressors shows that direct care workers who reported inadequate job orientation, mentoring, and continuing education programs had lower levels of job satisfaction (Menne, Noelker, Ejaz, & Fox, 2006). However, direct care workers' perceptions about the adequacy of their entry-level training had no effect, probably because most of the workers in this sample had been on the job for an average of almost 5 years, with their entry-level training far in the past. Among the job-related stressors, workers had lower job satisfaction scores when they perceived their continuing education sessions and mentors at time of hire as less useful. Clearly, the education and training of direct care workers has a significant impact on job satisfaction, which would be expected based on worker empowerment theory.

Other job-related stressors resulting in lower job satisfaction were direct care workers' complaints of management's failure to permanently assign residents to workers, reports that turnover among direct care workers was more stressful, and perceptions of compensation and benefits as inadequate. The presence of career ladders was not shown to have an effect on job satisfaction, probably because so few facilities had career advancement programs. Among workplace support factors, when workers reported less negative interaction in the workplace and fewer racist remarks directed at them by other staff, their job satisfaction scores were higher.

Analysis of the predictors of worker job satisfaction showed that their background characteristics such as age and marital status had no impact on job satisfaction. However, personal stressors also contributed to job dissatisfaction. Those who reported poorer self-rated physical health and more symptoms of depression had lower job satisfaction scores. Taken together, these findings underscore the importance of instituting workplace support systems that focus on alleviating or buffering the personal and job-related stress faced by direct care workers. The findings also underscore the importance of promoting good management practices, such as permanent assignment, as being pivotal to worker job satisfaction and are further evidence of the value of following workplace empowerment principles that enhance worker outcomes.

CONCLUSIONS

Findings from the research study provide recommendations for improving workplace practices that directly affect the empowerment of direct care workers. These include ways to improve training, job orientation, and continuing education. The findings also provide critical evidence about the value of higher-quality job orientation, mentoring, and continuing education programs for increased job satisfaction. Although perceptions of the value of entry-level training did not affect job satisfaction, this appeared to be related to the fact that, on average, direct care workers in the sample had been employed in the field for almost 5 years. Additionally, positive support in the workplace from coworkers and other staff was shown to attenuate the negative effects of personal and job-related stressors. Therefore, better, more extensive and intensive information that direct care workers perceive as necessary for the job, along with workplace support, are two of the essential components for worker empowerment and job satisfaction. Unfortunately, so few NHs in the study had career ladders that it was not possible to investigate direct care workers' perceptions about opportunities to learn and grow, a third key component of worker empowerment.

In the introduction to this chapter it was noted that innovations in education and training programs for direct care workers have been developed and evaluated recently, with promising results. For example, the LEAP (Learn, Empower, Achieve, Produce) program targets both direct care workers and their supervisors for advanced training around communication, teamwork, and leadership (Hollinger-Smith, Lindeman, Leary, & Ortigara, 2002; Hollinger-Smith, Ortigara, & Lindeman, 2001). Similarly, Workforce Improvement for Nursing Assistants: Supporting Training, Education, and Payment for Upgrading Performance (WIN A STEP UP) is a workforce development program for direct care workers in NHs that includes on-site continuing education, compensation for training, supervisory training, and payment for program completion (Craft, Morgan, & Conrad, 2007). Comparisons of nursing staff at participating and nonparticipating facilities showed that after 3 months, supervisors and direct care workers who received the training had higher team care scores and higher nursing care and supportive leadership scores.

Progress in the development and evaluation of new education and training programs and workplace interventions, such as the empowered work team, is pivotal in advancing the skill levels of the long-term care workforce and hence the quality of care they provide. In the course of program development, however, findings from this study point to the importance of involving direct care workers in planning their design and delivery. Furthermore, involving experienced direct care workers more in the training process and compensating them appropriately for this added responsibility were widely endorsed by direct care workers in this sample.

Acknowledgments

The chapter authors would like to thank the following funders and organizations for support of the research studies reviewed in this chapter: Cleveland Foundation, Retirement Research Foundation, Robert Wood Johnson Foundation, Atlantic Philanthropies, and the Institute for the Future of Aging Services at the American Association of Homes and Services for the Aging. We would also like to thank the project staff members who worked on these projects, including Kathleen Fox, Dorothy Schur, Julie Rentsch, and Justin Johnson, and the participating research sites, the respondents, and our interviewers.

PART III

Implementing Empowered Work Teams in Long-Term Care

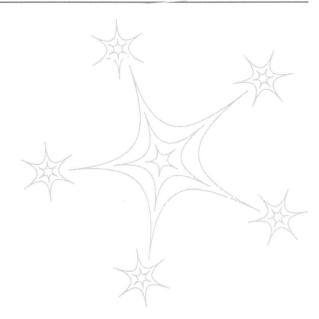

This part of the book is for those who want to implement empowered work teams (EWTs) in their organization. Time and care must be given to the implementation and maintenance of the teams in order to gain the benefits they can provide and avoid creating new problems.

The knowledge shared here on team implementation and maintenance comes primarily from experience in implementing 32 EWTs for direct care workers in six nursing homes (NHs) between 2002 and 2006. The first experience was with a 200-bed facility in east Dallas, Texas, where nine teams were created and more than 70 team meetings were either facilitated or observed. This first NH served as the pilot study for the empirical evaluation of EWTs described in Chapters 6 and 7. After this first experience, the implementation procedures were revised to take advantage of what was learned. The revised procedures were used to implement three teams in a 50-bed facility in Weatherford, Texas, a small city located roughly 60 miles west of Dallas. The implementation and team maintenance procedures were revised again, and four teams were implemented in a 110-bed facility in Denton, Texas, a midsized city. The procedures were again revised and then used to create four EWTs in a 120-bed facility in a suburb north of Dallas. The implementation procedures were improved further as 10 more EWTs were implemented in a 200-bed facility in Gunter, Texas, a rural area about 50 miles north of Dallas. Finally, the procedures described in this section were used to create two teams in a 50-bed facility in Fort Worth, Texas, serving a densely populated metropolitan area. In total, more than 390 team meetings were facilitated or observed. In addition, multiple meetings with the managers of each facility were held, as were training sessions for nurse managers, nurses, and direct care workers.

The lessons learned are incorporated into the chapters in this section. Chapter 9 focuses on the initial planning and staff orientation. Chapters 10 and 11 provide training materials for a variety of people involved with the EWTs, including nurse management, human resource personnel, nurses, EWT facilitators, team leaders, and EWT members. Chapter 12 reviews how to maintain the teams effectively. Finally, the steps for implementing EWTs in long-term care are listed in the Appendix.

CHAPTER 9

Initial Orientation for Empowered Work Teams

The first step in implementing empowered work teams (EWTs) is for several employees of your organization to gain familiarity with the concept. These people can then provide an initial orientation to managers and nurses that helps them to understand what EWTs are, their benefits, and their costs. This should be followed by an anonymous survey of the managers and nurses to determine whether they are open to the idea of empowering the direct care workers. If it appears that the managers and nurses are interested or at least open to the idea, then several people working within the organization should be selected to become experts on the topic, with the ability to provide staff orientation and training. These people must learn all that is available about EWTs, with a specific focus on EWTs used in your particular long-term care (LTC) setting, whether it is a nursing home (NH), assisted living facility, or home care provider. The initial orientation and planning are described in more detail in this chapter.

BECOMING FAMILIAR WITH THE CONCEPT OF EMPOWERED WORK TEAMS

In order to orient an organization's management and nurse staff to the concept of EWTs, it is necessary to have several staff people (or an outside source) who are familiar enough with the concept of EWTs to provide such an orientation. These people might include the administrator of the organization, director of nursing (DON), assistant director of nursing (ADON), or human resource manager. It is crucial that the selected people be open to the idea of empowering direct care workers or they will be unlikely to put forth the needed effort. These people should do an initial review of existing information to learn what EWTs are and how they work and to identify their strengths and weaknesses. This learning process might include reviewing existing literature on EWTs in LTC (e.g., Becker-Reems, 1994; Yeatts & Seward, 2000), attending conference sessions on the topic, and speaking with people who are involved with managing EWTs or who are EWT members.

An alternative (or in addition) to having several staff people become familiar with the topic is to invite someone from outside the organization to provide an orientation to the staff. This might include a staff person from a sister organization that is using EWTs or a consultant who has firsthand experience with EWTs. In either case, it is important that the person invited have firsthand or in-depth knowledge of such teams. Otherwise, she or he will not have the depth of knowledge needed to conduct an accurate orientation and answer staff questions.

INITIAL ORIENTATION FOR MANAGERS AND NURSES

It has been found that EWTs will not be successful unless the managers who supervise the employees are positive or at least neutral about empowering direct care workers such as certified nursing assistants (CNAs), universal workers, and home health aides. If managers or nurses are strongly opposed to EWTs, they may consciously or unconsciously do things to prevent the EWT from being successful. This usually takes the form of withholding (or forgetting to provide) information that the EWT needs in order to make good decisions, whether it is developing a new work process or identifying solutions to a problem. Therefore, it is extremely important that EWTs not be implemented unless the managers and nurses are in favor or at least not opposed to them.

To make this determination, provide all managers and nurses with an initial EWT orientation and then administer a short, anonymous questionnaire to obtain their views on EWTs. Those involved in the orientation should include all supervisors of direct care workers, such as the DON, ADON, and nurses as well as others who work with the direct care workers and residents, such as the activity director and social worker. Others might include the human resource manager, the financial officer, and department heads. The orientation should explain what EWTs are, their costs, and their benefits (see Exhibit 9A at the end of the chapter for a prepared presentation). More specifically, the following information should be provided to them (see Exhibit 9B at the end of the chapter):

- An EWT is a group of direct care workers, such as CNAs or home health aides, who work together daily and serve the same group of residents. The EWT reviews the health of residents, recommends solutions to problems, recommends new or revised work processes, and, as the team matures, provides input on decisions to be made by management and nurses.

- The benefits of EWTs have been found to include improved workplace decisions and processes and improved resident care. Improvements have been found to occur in part because of the firsthand knowledge that is obtained from the direct care workers. Furthermore, when direct care workers are involved in the development of new or revised work processes, the processes are more likely to be implemented successfully and continued over time. Studies have found that additional benefits to EWTs include more positive attitudes of both the direct care workers and nurses and lower turnover (see Chapter 7). Direct care workers who perceive themselves to be empowered in the workplace have been found to have much higher job satisfaction, commitment to the organization, and self-esteem and much lower job burnout (see Chapter 7).

- The cost of EWTs includes the time needed to train direct care workers, nurses, and managers; the time needed for EWT meetings in order to review the health of residents and develop recommendations regarding residents, work processes, and existing problems; the willingness among managers and supervisors to allow direct care workers to participate in decision making and to implement their suggestions; the time needed for the EWTs and nurse management to work together to finalize solutions or work processes; and implementation problems that must be overcome as the teams are forming (e.g., how the nurse management interacts with the EWTs).

SURVEYING MANAGERS AND NURSES

Once the managers and nurses have had a chance to consider what EWTs are, their benefits, and their costs, they should be surveyed to determine whether they think EWTs would work in their facility or organization (Exhibit 9C at the end of the chapter provides a brief survey instrument). The survey should be completely anonymous. This means that the personal responses of individuals can in no way be linked to them. This will increase the chance that the managers and nurses express their true opinions, not what they believe the administrator, DON, or other executive wants them to say. All those who would be involved in the day-to-day empowerment of the direct care workers should complete the survey, such as the DON, ADON, and nurses as well as the NH administrator.

At a minimum, these people should be asked the following:

- What two benefits they believe will result from EWTs and what two hindrances or costs. This will help to clarify how well they understand the concept of EWTs. If it is clear that some do not understand what EWTs are or how they work, then additional orientation should be provided to help clarify any misunderstandings.

- What they perceive to be the chances of EWTs being implemented successfully in their facility or organization. They should also be asked to explain their view. It is possible that their reasoning for the teams not working is a lack of information, and with more information they would change their opinion. On the other hand, the managers and nurses should not be made to feel that they are being pushed into changing their views of the potential for EWT success. If a majority or large minority do not believe that EWTs will be successful for any reason other than lack of understanding of what EWTs are, management would be wise not to implement EWTs.

- Whether they would like EWTs to be implemented in their facility or organization and the reasons for or against. In cases where there is general agreement against the use of EWTs, the reasoning of the managers and nurses will help to identify their thinking. If the negative opinion results from misinformation about EWTs or bad experiences in the past, then additional information about EWTs may be all that is needed to change their perspective. On the other hand, if additional information does not change management attitudes from negative to positive, then the implementation of EWTs should not proceed. Only when employees are open to the concept of empowered workers should EWTs be implemented.

Employee attitudes about EWTs provide some insight into your organization's culture. In addition to assessment of the level of interest in EWTs, a survey can determine the staff's view of the overall culture of the organization. A culture that is perceived to be friendly and open to new ideas from direct care workers is a culture where the implementation of EWTs is likely to succeed. A culture that is perceived to be hierarchical, with all decisions made strictly from the top, is not likely to provide the management or direct care worker support needed for successful implementation of EWTs.

Several organizations and individuals have developed in-depth survey instruments specifically for NH staffs to assess their existing organizational culture. Grant and Norton (2003) developed what they call a stage model of culture change for nursing facilities. Their survey instrument helps to identify how open the staff of an LTC facility is to sharing decision making, clarifies existing leadership practices, and examines the physical environment and staff roles. Also, the Institute for Caregiver Education has developed the Culture Change Indicators Survey, and the American College of Healthcare Administrators has developed the Leadership Assessment Survey.

It is interesting to note that in manufacturing settings, where EWTs have been used for decades, instruments to measure the views of managers and supervisors have been used by some but not others. Where they are used, organizations typically are concerned about whether a majority of their managers support the idea of empowering employees. In some organizations where it is found that a majority are not open to employee empowerment, a decision is made to withhold the implementation of EWTs until the managers and supervisors are more receptive. And this can take 5 years or more. In other organizations, the executives of the organization have been less patient or tolerant with the managers and supervisors opposed to EWTs. In these organizations, EWTs are implemented without a waiting period, and the managers and supervisors found to be resistant are either moved into nonsupervisory positions or released from the organization. This latter approach can be harsh for managers, and so it is recommended that the implementation of EWTs not occur until those who manage the direct care workers become comfortable with the concept of employee empowerment.

INITIAL ORIENTATION FOR DIRECT CARE WORKERS

It is best to take this step only after a decision has been made to go forward with EWTs. Providing the direct care workers with an orientation to EWTs and then not following through with implementation will greatly disappoint those who were particularly excited about the opportunity to participate in decisions related to their work.

The orientation of direct care workers should be similar to that provided to management and nurses (Exhibit 9A). This will include clarifying what an EWT is and describing its costs and benefits. Some direct care workers will be excited by this initiative and look forward to the opportunity to be more involved in the decisions related to their work. Still others may have been involved in empowerment initiatives that were successful in other organizations and so can help with the implementation process. On the other hand, some direct care workers will be more cautious in their enthusiasm, and still others will express a dislike for the idea. In the latter case, it is helpful to be aware of factors that can cause a negative reaction to the concept of EWTs.

A negative response to an EWT orientation may result from a direct care worker's previous experience where an EWT was implemented but proved to be unsuccessful. However, it is more likely that a negative response comes from the direct care workers' concerns that they will be unable to perform their new roles adequately. These workers typically are comfortable in their current role, knowing that they are successfully meeting their responsibilities. When new, untried responsibilities are introduced, these workers are unsure whether they will be able to continue being successful in their jobs. Consequently, they will resist change because it raises the risk of being unable to do the work and subsequently receiving poor evaluations. Similar employee viewpoints have been found where EWTs were being implemented in manufacturing settings.

Research on the implementation of EWTs in LTC settings (NHs more specifically) has shown that direct care workers who are initially pessimistic about EWTs eventually become some of the greatest supporters. For example, in one case a CNA had had a bad experience with work teams in a previous NH and wanted nothing to do with the initiation of EWTs in her current NH. The team facilitator did not insist that she participate in team meetings but only that she be present. As time progressed and the CNA observed the involvement of her coworkers, she found herself being drawn into discussions. As she became more and more involved over time, her fellow team members eventually encouraged her to take on the team leader role, which she did.

DEVELOPMENT OF SEVERAL EXPERTS ON EWTS

This step is taken if it is decided that EWTs will be implemented. The goal is to develop several people on the staff of the organization who will have knowledge beyond what EWTs are and how they work. These experts should be able to provide training to the managers, supervisors, nurses, and team members and to be an advocate for the team, particularly during implementation. An ideal person for this role is the organization's human resource manager. Others include the DON and the ADON. However, it is more important that the experts be people who strongly support the concept of empowering employees than it is to have experts who hold a particular job description. Otherwise, these experts will not provide the kind and level of training needed. For example, an ADON who questions whether CNAs can make good decisions is likely to provide supervisors and nurses with training that lacks encouragement for involving direct care workers in decision making. On the other hand, an ADON who believes in empowering direct care workers not only will encourage managers and nurses to involve direct care workers in decision making but also will provide training to the direct care workers that helps them make good decisions. Consequently, it is most important to select people who are in favor of EWTs and to avoid selecting people who are neutral about EWTs or who express an interest only because they know it will get them accolades from management or because they believe management wants them to do it.

The people who are to become experts on EWTs should begin by searching the literature and attending conference sessions that describe successful and unsuccessful EWTs in health care settings and other work settings. The references at the end of this book provide a good start on the existing literature. Because EWTs are also called self-managed work teams and self-directed work teams, literature searches and conference sessions should include these terms. Existing literature and conference sessions can help to clarify the factors that are most important to successful implementation and those that can inhibit or enhance EWT success. Literature can be obtained from associations and other organizations that encourage the empowerment of LTC workers (e.g., American Association of Homes and Services for the Aged, Institute for Caregiver Education, Paraprofessional Health Care Institute), from libraries, and directly from people who are more familiar with EWTs.

The next step is to contact and, where possible, visit people who work in similar organizations and have experience implementing and working with EWTs. This might include people in associations where EWTs have been encouraged (e.g., the American College of Healthcare Administrators, the National Clearinghouse on the Direct Care Workforce). Visits to an organization, such as an NH, that is using EWTs might include sitting in on an EWT meeting or speaking with an EWT leader or team members. Conversations and visits should center on issues such as the steps that were taken to implement the EWTs, the hurdles that had to be overcome before positive results emerged, how and when the teams meet to discuss issues, what kinds of decisions the EWTs are making, and the interactions that occur between management and the EWTs as recommendations are made.

CONCLUSION

Those who manage direct care workers must be willing to support the concepts of empowering employees and of EWTs. Therefore, surveying those who supervise direct care workers to determine their level of support is a prerequisite to team implementation. If the managers are open to the concept of EWTs, then several people in the organization can take on the task of learning all they can about EWTs and how to implement them. Once this is accomplished, they will be able to provide a thorough orientation to the direct care workers and develop training materials for managers, nurses, team facilitators, and direct care workers.

EXHIBIT 9A   Presentation Slides to Explain the Concept of EWTs

SLIDE 1

EWT = A GROUP OF DIRECT-CARE WORKERS (DCWS) WHO

- Serve the same group of residents
- Review the health of residents
- Recommend solutions to problems
- Recommend new or revised procedures
- Provide input on decisions to be made by management or nurses

SLIDE 2

WHY IMPLEMENT EWTS?

- Better workplace decisions
- Successful implemention and revision of work processes
- Improved resident care
- Improved DCW job attitudes
- Reduced turnover among DCWs

SLIDE 1 COMMENTARY

It is important for DCWs to realize that in an EWT they would be meeting together in order to consider how to improve work processes as well as to discuss the needs and preferences of the various residents. It is important that nurse managers recognize that the teams would need to be brought into the decision-making process.

Some concern may be expressed that at times a change in work process needs to be made relatively quickly so that there would be little time to consult the EWT. This is true. An appropriate response is that quickly made solutions are often not the best solutions. Quickly made solutions can be replaced later by more permanent solutions that have received EWT input.

SLIDE 2 COMMENTARY

Research has shown that the best decisions are made when the persons who actually do the work are involved in the decision-making process.

When the DCWs take part in decision making, they develop feelings of ownership. As a result, they are more willing to see the decisions actually implemented and then continued.

In addition to being used to make better workplace decisions, EWT meetings are used to review resident needs and preferences. This results in better resident care.

The results of better work processes and better care are less frustration and more satisfaction among the DCWs as well as among the DCWs and nurse management.

SLIDE 3

> COST = TIME
>
> - Time for training
>
> - Time for DCWs to evaluate a process or problem of concern
>
> - Time for DCWs to recommend a new process or solution as well as for management to receive, evaluate, and respond to DCW recommendations

SLIDE 3 COMMENTARY

The single most difficult requirement of EWTs is the time required of the DCWs.

The DCWs must make time to meet weekly to consider solutions to problems, discuss issues of concern, and review resident needs and preferences.

Nurse management must make time on a regular basis to involve the DCWs in decision making. This includes time for presenting issues to the EWT, evaluating the team's recommendations, providing feedback to the team, and reaching a solution that includes the EWT's input.

SLIDE 4

> MANAGERS MUST PLAN TIME TO
>
> - Provide information to the teams
>
> - Receive input from the teams
>
> - Consider team input
>
> - Respond in a positive way to the teams

SLIDE 4 COMMENTARY

In order for the EWTs to make good decisions, they must be given all of the relevant information needed. For example, when considering work processes for providing meals to residents, it would be helpful for the EWT to know the limitations of the kitchen staff in terms of when meals can be delivered.

If a decision made by the EWT needs to be returned to them for revision, it is still important to take time to recognize the team for the thought and effort they put into the decision.

SLIDE 5

MANAGERS MUST BE WILLING TO

- Allow participation in decision making

- Compromise

- Allow DCWs to make mistakes in decision making

SLIDE 5 COMMENTARY

In order for the EWTs to actually be "empowered," managers must be willing to allow the DCWs to either make decisions or at least to be involved in the decision-making process.

This can require nurse management to make compromises to their original solution in order to include the input from the EWT.

Nurse management can help the EWTs to become wiser in their decision making by allowing them to implement the decisions they propose, even when they appear to be poor decisions—as long as the decisions will not do any harm. In cases where the team proposes a poor solution and then implements it, the DCWs will eventually realize that they have implemented a poor solution and will move to correct it. In other cases, nurse management will learn from the team, discovering that what was thought to be a poor team choice has proven to be a good one.

SLIDE 6

IMPLEMENTATION PROBLEMS LIKELY TO OCCUR

- Some DCWs and managers will be unsure of their new responsibilities and will be concerned that they cannot perform them.

- Some DCWs and managers will by unhappy with a change or changes.

SLIDE 6 COMMENTARY

Some DCWs and nurse managers will fear that they lack the skills needed to either work within EWTs or to empower the EWTs. No doubt it does take trial and error, as everyone is learning their new responsibilities. Unless the DCWs and nurse managers are willing to put aside their fears and attempt to make the teams work, the EWTs should not be implemented.

In other cases, there will be DCWs who simply prefer not to be involved in decision making. They would prefer to just do what they are told and then go home. There will also be nurse managers who feel that they have worked for years to get to the stage where they can make the decisions. They do not want to include the input of DCWs. Other nurse managers may feel that the DCWs are not "smart enough" to identify the best decisions. It will be better not to implement EWTs unless a large majority of the DCWs and nurse managers support the idea of EWTs and are willing to give them a try.

SLIDE 7

> WHAT DO YOU SEE AS THE ADVANTAGES AND DIS-
> ADVANTAGES OF EMPOWERING OUR DCWS?

SLIDE 7 COMMENTARY

The primary purpose of this question is to help determine how well the DCWs and nurse managers understand the concept of EWTs, what it takes to make them work, and what their advantages are. If DCWs or managers mention advantages or disadvantages that should not be expected (e.g., DCWs will have longer breaks or DCWs will be doing the work of nurse managers), then they need further review of what an EWT is and how DCWs and nurse management will work together to make them successful.

SLIDE 8

> SURVEY OF ALL MANAGERS AND NURSES:
>
> • Are you open to empowering our DCWs? Will it help?
>
> (Survey is completely anonymous.)

SLIDE 8 COMMENTARY

At this point, the DCWs and nurse managers should be informed that there will be an anonymous survey. The questionnaire will allow them the opportunity to voice their anonymous opinion as to whether EWTs should be implemented. No one will know how others answered. Everyone's answers will be aggregated and, unless a large majority of the DCWs and nurse managers want to implement EWTs, they will not be implemented. It is entirely up to the DCWs and nurse management since EWTs cannot be successfully implemented unless they want them to work. A sample questionnaire that could be used is provided on page 132 of this book.

Three Commonly Asked Questions About Empowered Work Teams (and Their Answers)

WHY CREATE EWTS?

- People who are allowed to make decisions about their work feel better about their work, are more motivated to carry out the decisions made, and feel more responsible for making sure the decisions are carried out than when procedures are dictated to them. For example, if an EWT is involved in deciding how resident call lights are handled, team members will be more motivated and committed to making sure the decision is carried out.

- EWTs are able to identify where problems are in the work process and identify meaningful solutions or new ways of doing things that improve the work process.

- The nursing staff may be able to save time by allowing the EWT to make certain decisions.

- Over time, teams can help the direct care workers build trust and collegiality with one another and with the nursing staff.

WHAT DECISIONS WILL THE EWTS MAKE?

- In some cases the teams will be asked by managers or nurses to make a specific workplace decision such as how to best assist residents into the dining room when they are short staffed.

- In other cases EWTs may be asked simply to provide their input on a decision to be made, such as how to handle a particular resident who has become combative.

- In still other cases, the EWT may come to a manager or nurse and ask for permission to begin making a particular decision, such as the daily assignment of residents to direct care workers.

HOW WILL MY JOB CHANGE AS A RESULT OF EWTS BEING USED?

- If you are a nurse or manager, you will be expected to either solicit the opinion of the team before making decisions that involve the team, make a joint decision with the team by together considering possible solutions, or allow the team to make a decision that you had been making before the team was created.

- If you are a direct care worker, you will be expected to work with other direct care workers on your team to provide input before a nurse or manager makes a decision, or make a joint decision with a nurse or manager by together considering possible solutions, or make a team decision and then, with nurse or management approval, implement it.

Are Empowered Work Teams Right for Our Organization?

Please provide your thoughts about establishing empowered work teams in our facility. Your answers will be completely anonymous. Do not put your name on this sheet or write anything that will identify you.

1. List two benefits you believe will result from using empowered work teams.

2. List two hindrances or costs to using empowered work teams.

3. What are the chances that empowered work teams will work in our facility? (circle one)

No Chance   Will Definitely Work

   0   10   20   30   40   50   60   70   80   90   100

Please explain:

4. Do you personally want to see empowered work teams established in our facility? (circle one)

                        No   Not Sure   Yes

Please explain:

CHAPTER 10

Training Managers and Nurses for Empowered Work Teams in Long-Term Care

In order for empowered work teams (EWTs) to be successful, the team members need to know how to meet together, discuss the health of residents, consider alternative work procedures, investigate work-related problems, and make effective decisions. The team facilitator must have the knowledge to assist the team members in developing the skills needed to accomplish these tasks. The nurses and managers of the organization need to learn how to involve EWTs in decision making, particularly decisions related to resident care and work procedures. And the human resource (HR) director must be able to orient new employees, such as nurses and direct care workers, to the concept of EWTs. Clearly, the knowledge and skills needed are quite extensive. The purpose of the next two chapters is to provide in-house trainers with information they can use to develop their own training materials for all those who will receive training, including managers, nurses, team members, team facilitators, team leaders, and HR personnel.

It is important to note several training tips related to training empowered direct care workers, nurses, and managers. First, the timing of the training should occur within a few days or at most several weeks before the direct care workers, nurses, and managers will practice what they are being taught. Managers and nurses are likely to be negligent in involving direct care workers in decision making if they are shown how to involve EWTs in decision making but then asked not to do so for several weeks or months. Direct care workers will become frustrated if they are taught how to participate in decision making and to solve problems but then are not allowed to practice this new ability for weeks or months.

Second, it is important that the trainer not get the direct care workers too excited about their new decision-making responsibilities. Trainers will want to gain buy-in from the direct care workers so that they will put forth the effort needed to meet weekly, discuss resident issues, solve problems, develop improved procedures, and so on. One way to gain buy-in is to emphasize the decision-making authority that the direct care workers will have. However, if the trainer focuses on this too much, the team members will be greatly disappointed if they discover that the nurses and managers are going to allow them to make few decisions or to have minimal input into decision making initially.

Third, it is important that the trainers not attempt to implement too many EWTs at one time. Experience shows that each EWT will need a good deal of time from nurse management and nurses as the team learns how to meet as a team, consider issues, and ask management and nurses for feedback. Implementing more

133

than two EWTs at one time can overburden nurse management to the point that the teams do not receive the attention and positive feedback they need from the director of nursing (DON) and assistant director of nursing (ADON).

SELECTING AND TRAINING THE TRAINERS

Those providing training for the implementation of EWTs can be current employees of the long-term care (LTC) organization or trainers external to the organization. As noted in Chapter 9, the job titles of the people who provide the training are not as important as the commitment of the people to creating effective EWTs. Perhaps the most important characteristics to consider when selecting the trainers are their belief and confidence in the empowerment of direct care workers. Some people naturally want to empower those around them, including direct care workers. Others have a basic belief that direct care workers should not be involved in management issues. Reasons can vary from a desire not to burden the direct care worker with management decision making to a belief that direct care workers do not have the necessary intellect, education, maturity, and so on. If the trainer has any doubts about the ability of direct care workers to contribute to management decision making or to work effectively in EWTs, then the trainer will be less effective than she or he could be.

Also noted in Chapter 9, the people selected to be the trainers will need to conduct a literature review on EWTs in LTC (including reading this book), attend conferences on the subject, and speak with EWT members and people working with and managing EWTs to learn their perceptions of what it takes to be successful. They must use these sources to gain a good understanding of EWTs, including their advantages, costs, and uses, what the teams can do, and how the teams should interact with nurse management. Chapters 2–4 describe EWT–management interactions in nursing homes (NHs), assisted living facilities, and home care organizations, respectively. Ideally, the trainers will have already had the experience of orienting the managers, nurses, and direct care workers to the uses of EWTs. From this experience it will be a natural extension to provide more in-depth training to these groups.

TRAINING MANAGERS AND NURSES

This training should be targeted to the managers, supervisors of direct care workers, and other nurses who have traditionally made the decisions related to the work of direct care workers, particularly the procedures they use for doing the work (e.g., the procedures followed for getting residents up in the morning or performing a home care visit). The managers and nurses must be trained to recognize the workplace decisions that can be handed off to the EWTs, recognize the workplace decisions that could benefit from EWT input, provide EWTs with the information they need to make good decisions, successfully hand off decision making or request EWT input, and listen, communicate, and receive decisions or input from the EWTs. More specifically, regardless of whether the managers and nurses decide simply to ask for input or allow the EWTs to make decisions, the most important step is to get the EWTs involved in the decisions and to respect the input provided. This requires that the EWTs be given the information they need to make the best decision or recommendation. It also means communicating with the EWTs and being open to whatever the EWTs decide or recommend.

First Training Session

The first training session should begin with a brief review of the orientation previously provided. This includes a brief description of what EWTs are, their purpose, their costs (particularly time demands), and their benefits (see Chapter 9, Exhibit 9A, for a prepared orientation). This brief review can then be followed by a more detailed presentation of the team's purpose and responsibilities, how the teams will carry them out, and a review of management's responsibilities related to the teams:

Team Purpose

- To improve resident care

- To improve direct care worker work attitudes

- To reduce turnover and absenteeism

Team Responsibilities

- *Conduct a weekly review of the health of all residents* that the EWT serves, identify any concerns that must be shared with the nurse management (e.g., a resident has difficulty swallowing, a resident is more confused than normal), and make recommendations about the residents of concern. For example, a team member may report in an EWT meeting that a particular resident appears to be developing a bed sore. The team would discuss what appears to be causing the sore and what might be done to eliminate it. This information would then be passed on to nurse management.

- *Respond to requests from nurse management.* Nurse management may identify a problem that needs to be solved and ask the team to review the problem and provide a viable solution. For example, nurse management may report to the EWT that when residents request assistance they sometimes have to ask for help more than once. The team is given the responsibility of determining what is causing this problem and offering a viable solution. Or a manager or nurse may request that the team develop a new process for getting residents up in the morning or request that the team prepare a brief description of each resident's likes and dislikes that would then be made available to new or temporary direct care workers.

- *Provide input on decisions to be made by management or nurses.* The EWT may be asked to consider something of importance to management or nurses and provide its views on the issue. Issues of importance could range from the time at which a particular shift should start to a consideration of which food brand to offer to residents.

- *Recommend new or revised procedures.* Nurse management may want to try something new or perhaps has obtained new equipment that must be incorporated into the delivery of service. In such cases, nurse management may ask the EWT to develop and recommend procedures that incorporate the new ideas or new technology. Or nurse management may conclude that particular procedures being used are less than satisfactory and ask the EWT to develop more effective procedures. Likewise, on its own initiative, the EWT may conclude that particular procedures being used are less than effective and suggest that alternative procedures be used.

- *Report issues of EWT concern to management or nurses* and make recommendations as needed. The team should discuss workplace issues of concern to team members as they arise and either solve the issue within the team or report it to nurse management. For example, the direct care workers may be concerned that they are unable to take scheduled breaks because of their job demands. The team may choose to develop a solution and present it to management and nurses or simply report their concern and ask for help in solving the problem. Or the EWT may be having difficulty assisting residents in a timely manner during mealtime using existing procedures and may request the opportunity to consider alternative procedures or simply recommend alternative procedures.

- *Be sensitive to the feelings of other team members during team discussions.* Although there can and will be disagreements, all team member opinions should be respected. That is, if two team members disagree, each must be sure to respect the opinion of the other.

- *More mature teams* can be responsible for peer (team member) evaluations, evaluations of management and nurses, and interviews of direct care worker candidates who are applying to be members of the EWT.

Team Procedures

- *EWTs hold weekly 30-minute sit-down meetings* to carry out their responsibilities. During these team meetings, an agenda is followed that helps the team to achieve its goals (see Chapter 11, Exhibit 11A).

- *A team notebook is maintained* that includes a page for each team meeting reporting who was at the meeting and what items were reviewed and discussed (see Chapter 11, Exhibit 11B). This page is a means for the team to report any resident or direct care worker concerns to nurse management. It also provides space for nurse management to respond to direct care worker concerns.

- *EWTs hold short stand-up meetings* to make on-the-spot decisions (e.g., how to get immediate work done after a direct care worker becomes ill or injured while at work).

Management Responsibilities

- *Time must be provided for the team to meet each week.* The team will need roughly 30 minutes at least once a week to accomplish its weekly agenda and address any issues provided by management and nurses. Once the team has established a set day and time to meet each week, someone will need to take care of the residents' needs while team members are meeting. This typically means that the nurses will need to cover for the direct care workers during the meeting. Attempts have been made to avoid this hardship on the nurses by having the teams meet before or after their regular shift. However, in many cases this has caused hardships for direct care workers who have obligations just before or after their shifts, such as dropping a spouse off somewhere before coming to work or picking up children immediately after work. Consequently, careful consideration should be given to scheduling team meetings.

- *Someone must help the team facilitator and team leader make sure all team members attend the meetings.* This person typically is the team's supervisor or the ADON or DON. Many direct care workers will need encouragement to attend the team meetings. Typically, direct care workers have difficulty completing all of their tasks in the time available. Taking time for a meeting only makes it more difficult to satisfy all of the residents' needs. A supervisor should provide encouragement and arrange for someone to cover for the direct care workers (e.g., answer resident call lights) during the weekly team meeting.

- *Someone must take responsibility for working with the teams and responding to weekly team notes.* This person typically is a supervisor of the direct care workers, an ADON, or the DON. The direct care workers will review a variety of topics during their team meeting. Notes of the meeting are recorded and passed on to this person. This person reads the notes, confers with appropriate personnel (e.g., DON, housecleaning manager, food service manager) and then gives feedback to the EWTs.

- *When appropriate, give the teams an opportunity to make decisions about their work,* provide them with the information they need to make the best decision, and provide feedback on the decisions made. Here it is important to give the teams enough time and the appropriate information to make good decisions. The teams are trained to use a rational choice method for decision making that relies on generating and considering several possible alternatives and then selecting the best one (see Chapter 11). If the team is asked to make a decision without time to thoroughly consider alternatives, it is unrealistic to expect the team members to make the best, most considered decision. Although sometimes this is unavoidable, such decisions often result in "satisficing," or selecting an alternative that meets a minimal standard but is not necessarily the best alternative possible. Consequently, if a decision must be made immediately, it is advisable that managers ask the team to make a temporary decision immediately and later spend time identifying and selecting the best alternative.

An example can illustrate the importance of providing all relevant information. In one case, an EWT spent several hours poring over alternatives before finally reporting back to nurse management what the team concluded was the best choice. Nurse management then showed the team that this was not the best alternative available by presenting them with information that had never been shared with the team before. This resulted in the team members concluding that management "was going to do what they wanted to anyway." Furthermore, the team members concluded that in the future they would not take such requests from management seriously.

- *Management and nurse support of the teams and the decisions they make is crucial.* If a manager or nurse disregards the team's choice because it is not what the manager or nurse believes was the best choice, then the team members will be less motivated to identify alternatives and weigh strengths and weaknesses because they will believe that the alternative they select will be rejected by management anyway. Consequently, it is advisable to allow teams to make wrong choices and learn from them, except when the wrong choice would have negative impacts on residents.

Management Procedures

- *On a weekly basis, read the EWT notebook and respond to any concerns, issues, or comments of the direct care workers* in a timely fashion (i.e., don't wait several weeks to respond to the team's weekly notes).

- *When desiring input or a decision from the team, meet with the EWT to describe in detail what is desired* and provide the EWT with all the information needed so it can make a good decision or provide meaningful input.

- *In many cases nurse management must make a decision or revise existing procedures* before the EWT has time to make its own decision or develop new procedures (e.g., the health care department gives the NH only a short period of time to revise a particular procedure, or a resident complaint must be responded to immediately). In these cases, the EWT or nurse management should make a temporary decision or develop temporary procedures and then replace the temporary solution with the team's permanent solution once the team has had time to work with nurse management on the issue.

Subsequent Training Session: Use of Scenarios

Once management and the nurses have a basic understanding of their and the team's responsibilities and procedures, they will be ready to consider in more detail how to interact with the team. One valuable method is to provide managers, nurses, and direct care workers with scenarios that they might encounter (see Exhibit 10A at the end of the chapter for several scenarios).

Subsequent Training Session: Communicating with Teams

It is important that management and nurses have open and continuous communication with the EWTs. This means that the teams are continually provided information about the workplace and are aware and involved in the decisions being made. Unfortunately, involving the teams in decision making takes time. On the other hand, a major payoff is that the decisions made are likely to be practiced for a long period of time because those carrying out the decisions (the direct care workers) have had meaningful input. Likewise, the disadvantage of not involving the teams is that the decisions made are likely to be ignored by those carrying them out once management and the nurses turn their attention to other things.

Working with the EWTs to develop a decision that management, nurses, and the EWTs are all satisfied with typically is not easy. It takes multiple exchanges of ideas and compromise to reach a solution that everyone can tolerate. Of course, management and the nurses can force their opinions or decisions on the EWTs, so perhaps compromising is tougher for them because it is easy to simply decide that a particular decision has been made.

Play ball is a term that was created by trainers in the industrial setting to reflect the kind of successful interaction that can occur between the EWT and managers and supervisors. It reflects the process whereby the team provides suggestions to the managers or supervisors, who then provide feedback to the team, with the team providing modified suggestions in turn, and so on, until a final decision is reached. For example, an NH team may have learned from the DON that a number of residents and their family members have complained that breakfast trays are not delivered in a timely manner so that food is cold when it is served. The DON asks the team to develop a more efficient process for passing out trays. The team meets and follows prescribed problem-solving steps (see Chapter 11, Exhibit 11C). The solution selected is then "thrown back" to the DON, who evaluates it. The DON may accept the EWT solution as is, may develop some changes to it, or may note serious shortcomings of the solution. Once she or he decides how to respond to the EWT, the DON "throws" a response back to the team. In cases where the DON reports a serious shortcoming in the EWT's solution, the EWT typically lacks some crucial information, causing the design of their solution to be unworkable. In the case of handing out food trays, the team may have lacked crucial information on how early the food can be delivered or how much the food service staff can be expected to do. The DON must take responsibility, when throwing back her response, for providing the EWT with the information it is lacking and then allow the team members to reassess their solution with this additional information in hand. This "play ball" process shows ideas and possible solutions being thrown back and forth between the team and a management or nursing staff person until all agree on the solution to be adopted.

Subsequent Training Session: Offering a Team Excellence Award

Offering a team excellence award can have many positive results, although care must be taken to avoid negative effects that can also occur. A team excellence award can be used to clarify what management and nurses are looking for from the teams. It can also be used to encourage the direct care workers to meet on a regular basis and carry out their responsibilities. And it can heighten the direct care workers' interest in working on a team and can help the direct care workers see that management and nurses are sincere in their desire to involve the EWTs in decision making.

Exhibit 10B provides sample requirements for a team excellence award for teams that have just started meeting. In this case, the award emphasizes the importance of meeting regularly, taking notes of team activities, and getting the notes to the proper managers. The team awards can range from monetary prizes, to coupons for a free movie, to simple acknowledgment of the good work of a particular EWT at an all-staff meeting.

A major negative effect that has been recognized in manufacturing settings is the competition that can arise between teams. Although this can be positive if each team is trying to perform at a higher level than the other, it can be negative if the teams come to the point of not working well together. We did not find this to be a problem in the NH setting, but it would be wise to watch how the teams are responding to the award. Be sure that the teams are showing the kinds of behavior being sought and not also practicing less desirable behaviors.

Subsequent Training Session: Recognizing Stages of Team Development

It is important that the trainer help management and nurses recognize that the EWTs can be expected to move through at least four stages of development, with periodic movements back and forth between stages even after the fourth, "performing" stage, is reached. This will help the managers and nurses to better understand the behavior of the teams. These four stages—forming, storming, norming, and performing—have been identified by organizational researchers and our own

---

EXHIBIT 10B.
Sample Requirements for Obtaining a Team Excellence Award ($25 for each team member)

---

1. The team must meet 6 weeks in a row for first $25 and 10 weeks in a row for second $25. If for some reason the team cannot meet on its regular day, it should pick a different day in the week to meet.

2. The team needs to have a person who will fill in when the team leader is not at work on the meeting day.

3. Someone on the team must take notes during meeting. These should include the following:

   • Review of agenda items covered during the meeting

   • Any other issues covered and important to team members

   • Team response to notes received from the director of nursing or others

4. A copy of the team notes must be placed in the director of nursing's box or in the box of whomever management has selected to receive and review team notes.

---

experiences in LTC (Becker-Reems, 1994, provides a thorough discussion of these stages).

1. *Forming.* At this first stage of development, direct care workers are brought together and begin meeting regularly as a team. It is at this point that team members begin asking, "Why are we meeting?" "What is the purpose of the team?" The direct care workers begin discovering which team members support the idea of EWTs and which are less supportive. They are learning who is willing to take on a leadership role and who is willing to put forth effort to help the team succeed. At this stage it is important that a clear agenda be provided to the EWT. Otherwise, the team can be expected to develop its own agenda, which typically will include wage and staffing issues (e.g., a request for higher wages and more direct care workers on their shift). Therefore, it is important that the teams understand what issues they are to focus on and how they are to participate in decision making.

2. *Storming.* At this stage the team members have begun sharing their ideas with each other but have not yet learned how to communicate well or to reach compromises or consensus. They are learning which direct care workers view the work environment as they do and which have very different views of the work. In her study of health care organizations, Becker-Reems (1994, p. 159) found that "one of the most common causes of a team entering this stage is when one team member believes that he or she has been betrayed by another team member. The betrayal may be in the form of gossip, failure to support, failure to endorse ideas, or failure to show respect." Such disagreements can result in stormy relationships, with some direct care workers deciding they no longer trust or respect certain others or they no longer want to be on the team. It is at this stage that management and nurses may feel that the teams are failing and should be discontinued.

3. *Norming.* At this stage group members have become more settled and comfortable with working together, have established norms for their team meetings and other activities, and have begun to feel cohesiveness as a group. This stage typically follows the storming stage because team members are exhausted from all the interpersonal conflict and disruptions and are ready to establish a truce. Subsequently, norms are informally agreed upon, and team members attempt to maintain them. The primary concern here is that in order to avoid conflict, the team will not always consider a variety of competing ideas when seeking the best solution to a problem. For example, the team may be asked to identify an effective procedure for answering resident call lights. At the team meeting, one of the direct care workers may suggest a procedure, and then everyone else will choose to agree in order to get along and avoid conflict. Meanwhile, one or more team members may actually know of a more effective procedure but choose not to rock the boat by suggesting it. This has been called groupthink, in which all the team members accede to the first suggestion made in order to maintain peace and avoid conflict. Following the

Steps for Finding a Solution to a Current Problem (Exhibit 11C) will help to avoid this problem.

4. *Performing*. At this stage the group of direct care workers has become a highly functional team. They have learned how to make the most of their team meetings, practice cooperative conflict (see Chapter 11), and identify the most effective solutions to problems. The new ways of working as a team are now familiar and have become routine. Team members feel positive about their team and its ability to participate in the decision-making process. A key to success here is to keep the team engaged in decision making. If the team is not routinely provided new decision-making challenges, the direct care workers will lose their enthusiasm and may begin to question the value of the team or may fall back to a storming stage.

Subsequent Training Session: An Overview of the Training that the Teams, Team Facilitators, Team Leaders, and Human Resource Staff Are Receiving

The managers and nurses should be provided an overview of the training other employees are receiving. This will teach them what is being expected of these other employees and what the other employees will expect of the managers and nurses.

TRAINING HUMAN RESOURCE DIRECTORS

It is important that HR directors understand the skills that make EWTs successful. This includes the interpersonal skills and mindset that managers and nurses will need in order to involve the EWTs in decision making and the interpersonal and problem-solving skills that direct care workers will need to accomplish their goals. Responsibilities of the HR director related to the EWTs include the following:

- Hiring new staff who have experience with EWTs or are open to the use of EWTs and who either have the skills needed or are open to obtaining the skills needed to foster successful EWTs (see Exhibit 10C at the end of the chapter).

- Providing an orientation for newly hired managers, nurses, and direct care workers so they understand the value of the teams and the responsibilities of the direct care workers, managers, and nurses as they relate to the EWTs. This can be accomplished by using the orientation materials discussed earlier when first orienting staff to EWTs or by having the trainer meet with the newly hired people to provide an orientation.

- Helping the trainers identify potential training materials, as described earlier, that will enhance EWT success. These could be training modules focused on communication, cooperative conflict, interpersonal relations, problem solving, and so on. They might also include identification of conferences and consultants who could be of help.

In order to carry out these responsibilities, the HR director will need to understand how the EWTs function, understand how they interact with management and nurses, and be aware of the variety of skills needed for success. If the HR director is serving as the trainer for the direct care workers, managers, and nurses, then she or he should follow the training suggestions described earlier for trainers. If not, it will be important for the HR director to understand the relationship between the EWTs and managers and nurses and to learn what skills managers, nurses, and direct care workers need for EWT success. This can be accomplished by attending the training for managers and nurses and for direct care workers and noting the variety of skills needed or by consulting with the trainers. It would also be beneficial to attend some EWT meetings and attend meetings where the EWT is meeting with managers or nurses in the process of solving a problem or revising a work procedure.

Training for the successful implementation of EWTs, therefore, involves all levels of staff and management in a care facility. The next chapters describe in detail the training needed by the direct care workers who form the heart of EWTs.

Scenarios to Help Managers and Nurses Work with EWTs

Provided here are scenarios that managers and nurses might encounter. Situations are presented along with ways of responding that will encourage the EWTs. During a busy work day it is difficult to respond to teams in a well-thought-out way. These scenarios can help managers and nurses think through how they want to respond so that when the time comes they will have already thought through how to respond and be as supportive as possible.

1. **Management has decided that the nursing home needs to implement a hydration program. How would you involve the EWTs in helping to develop this program?**

After the managers and nurses have discussed how this might be done, present to them the following steps.

   1. *Let the direct care workers know* about the need for a hydration program (i.e., why there is a need and what has brought this on).

   2. *Ask the direct care workers to develop a hydration program* for distributing water to residents. Their program should detail how the program would work.

   3. *Give the direct care workers time* to develop a program during their weekly meetings.

   4. Once the EWT makes its initial proposal, *consider the proposed hydration program*.

   5. *Modify the proposed program if necessary* and then give it back to the EWT for its review and comment. Obtain the team's response to the modifications and seriously consider any additional modifications that it suggests.

   6. *Provide a description of the finalized program* to the EWT. The team members can pass on the description to any team members who were absent the day the program description was provided.

   7. Ask the teams to *evaluate* the program's implementation and operation after it has been in effect for a week or so.

   8. *Make adjustments* to the program based on the team's evaluation; be sure not to ignore its evaluation.

   In this scenario, gaining the teams' buy-in will ensure that the program is actually implemented and maintained. How often are great programs developed and started but then fall by the wayside as soon as management and nurses turn their attention to other issues? If the teams buy in to the program, the direct care workers will take ownership and maintain the program over time. Consequently management will not constantly be fighting with the direct care workers to carry out the program. How do managers and nurses gain direct care worker buy-in? They must seriously listen to the EWTs during the program's development and modify the program based on team input and later evaluations.

2. **You notice that a team's procedures for giving residents showers are not working well for some of the residents and their families. How can you involve the teams in correcting this problem?**

After the managers and nurses have discussed how this might be done, have them consider the following steps:

1. When the manager or nurse first observes the problem, *pitch in and help* the direct care workers so that the immediate problem is taken care of (if you are short on time, find some additional help for the direct care workers).

2. *Call a brief team meeting* and explain that you have observed that the procedures for giving residents showers do not seem to be working well for some of the residents and their families. Be sure to describe what is not working for the residents and their families.

3. *Ask the direct care workers about these problems.* If they answer, "The problem is normally avoided," ask them to consider, in their next team meeting, why their normal procedures are not always followed and then develop recommendations that will ensure that the procedures can always be followed.

4. If the team answers, "The problem you describe is not usually avoided with the procedures we use," *ask them to come up with a temporary solution* so that the problem does not continue and then to develop a permanent solution at their next team meeting that they will share with management.

3. **You have learned of a procedure that is being used in another facility or organization that seems to be having very positive outcomes. You want to implement the procedure in your organization. How can you use the teams to help you do this?**

After the managers and nurses have discussed how this might be done, have them consider the following steps:

1. *Describe the program and its advantages to the teams.* Ask the teams to list the pros and cons of implementing it at your nursing home.

2. *Review the teams' comments.*

3. *Ask the teams to redesign the program* so that it addresses their concerns.

4. *Consider the redesigns provided by the teams* and from these develop a design that meets as many of the teams' concerns as possible.

5. *Provide the teams with a description of the revised program* and explain that it tries to incorporate team concerns. Ask them for additional input.

6. *Make additional revisions based on their comments* and then ask the teams to implement the program with the understanding that it will be evaluated after being in operation for a few weeks.

7. After a few weeks, *ask the teams to provide feedback on the implementation and operation of the program.*

8. *Revise the program based on team input.*

It is a good idea to avoid implementing too many different programs over a short span of time. Give the teams time to adjust to one change before implementing another. Al-

(continued)

though these steps will take what seems to be a tremendous amount of time, consider the following: Do you want a program that you implement to continue only until you turn your attention to something else? Or do you want a program that, once implemented and evaluated, will continue to operate long after you have turned your attention to other concerns?

4.   **A team wants to implement a new procedure for caring for difficult residents. They come to you with their idea. How do you respond?**

After the managers and nurses have discussed how this might be done, have them consider the following steps:

1.   *Ask the team to describe what they are doing* to deal with difficult residents and how the new procedure differs from this.

2.   *Ask them for time* to review their proposed program but explain that you will respond in a timely fashion (e.g., within a week).

3.   *Consider the pros and cons* of their program.

*   *If the cons are not serious,* allow the teams to implement the program and ask them to give you a report on its strengths and weaknesses after they have been using it for awhile.

*   *If there are some serious concerns* or the cons appear to clearly outweigh the advantages of the proposed program, go back to the team and describe for them what you see as the problems with the proposed program. Ask them to modify their proposed program so that it will avoid the identified problems. Once they have done this, they can present it to you again so that you can reconsider it.

4.   If the program has been modified and resubmitted to you, *reconsider the pros and cons of the program*. If the serious concerns have been eliminated, allow the team to implement the program. If not, go back to the team and describe for them what you still see to be major concerns with the proposed program.

5.   **Absenteeism has become an increasing problem and you want to find a way to lower it. How can the teams help?**

After the managers and nurses have discussed how this might be done, have them consider the following steps:

1.   *Explain the problem* to the teams and ask them to come up with some ways to avoid the problem (experience facilitating EWTs has shown that the teams have a variety of ideas for reducing absenteeism that appear to be reasonable and would work if implemented).

2.   *If the teams present a sound plan to reduce absenteeism,* implement the plan on at least one floor and ask the EWTs to evaluate it.

3.   If you find that a combination of ideas from the various teams can be used to produce what appears to be the best plan, *present this new plan to the teams* and ask

them to consider the pros and cons at their next team meeting and then present them to you.

4. Based on team input, *modify the plan* and then go back to the teams, describe the modifications, and ask for additional input.

5. After further consideration of input, *provide further modification to the plan* with an attempt to satisfy the concerns of the teams, even if it does not seem to be the best approach.

6. *Implement the plan* with the understanding that the teams will be asked to evaluate it after using it for a few months.

Nurse management has two choices: It can either take only the best of what the teams offer, develop the plan, and ask the teams to implement it. Or management can take all of what the teams offer except for what clearly would be destructive, develop the plan, and ask the teams to implement it. Experience shows that the teams are much more likely to implement and continue to use the plan if all their ideas are used, not just those that seem best to management. After their ideas are implemented, if some of them do not work, the teams will discover this and then be ready to implement something else. However, if they do not have the opportunity to learn that their proposed ideas will not work, they will still want to implement them. Therefore, you will increase the chances of having the plan implemented and permanently in place by designing it to include the teams' suggestions even if the suggestions do not seem to be the best.

Information for Newly Hired Direct Care Workers About the Organization's Empowered Work Teams

- Direct care workers have been organized into empowered work teams (EWTs).

- You will work on one of these teams, depending on which shift you work and which floor or hall you work on.

- Each EWT has a sit-down meeting once a week for roughly 30 minutes and has short stand-up meetings as needed.

- The purpose of the sit-down meetings is to give the direct care workers an opportunity to discuss their work among themselves, give each other updates on the residents, improve work processes (such as the process of handing out meal trays or getting residents up in the morning), and assist each other with any problems that arise.

- The team meetings are led by one of the team members, and only team members and the team facilitator attend the meetings.

- Each team has a notebook. At each team meeting one of the team members writes down what was discussed at the meeting, such as the condition of the residents reviewed, discussions about the work process, and issues of concern to the direct care workers. The notes are then read by nurse management, who often provide feedback that is read by the team at its next meeting.

- An agenda is provided to the direct care workers for their team meetings. The agenda reminds the direct care workers to discuss the health of residents, any work procedures that need attention, and any others issues as they come up.

CHAPTER 11

Training Direct Care Workers for Empowered Work Teams in Long-Term Care

Direct care worker training should be targeted to employees working in an empowered work team (EWT). They typically include certified nursing assistants in a nursing home (NH) or assisted living facility and home care workers or universal workers in home care organizations. These direct care workers must be trained to meet together in both sit-down and stand-up meetings, provide routine information about the residents to management and nurses, make workplace decisions and develop new programs and plans as requested by management and nurses, report direct care worker concerns to management and the nurses as they arise, and listen, communicate, and receive feedback or decisions from management and nurses. More specifically, regardless of whether the managers and nurses decide simply to ask for input or allow the EWTs to make decisions, the most important step is for the EWTs to become involved in the decisions and make well-considered recommendations as requested by management and nurses. This means using problem-solving techniques, communicating regularly with management and the nurses, and being open to the modifications to team recommendations suggested by management and nurses.

FIRST TRAINING SESSION

The first training session should begin with a brief review of the orientation previously provided to the direct care workers. This includes a brief description of what EWTs are, their purpose, their costs (particularly time demands), and their benefits (see Chapter 9, Exhibit 9A, for a prepared orientation). This brief review can be followed by a more detailed presentation of the team's purpose and responsibilities, an explanation of how the teams will carry these out, and a review of management's responsibilities related to the teams. Chapter 10 provides details regarding management, nurse, and EWT responsibilities, which will not be repeated here. Nevertheless, the direct care workers should be provided training that covers the same materials.

SUBSEQUENT TRAINING SESSION: THE TEAM MEETING

The direct care workers should have an understanding of their new responsibilities and be aware that team meetings are to be used as a primary means of accomplishing them. A separate training session can be provided to review exactly how the team meetings are to operate and to determine the logistics related to the meetings. Ideally, this training would be provided individually for each team, with the team's facilitator also present during the training.

The team can begin this session by making one of its first decisions: when and where it will hold its team meetings. Teams typically want to hold their meeting at a time of the day when their duties are lightest. This might be near the end of their shift, when residents have finished their meals and are taking a nap (day shift) or have gone to bed for the night (evening shift). Sometimes teams want to meet the last half hour of their shift and then encourage direct care workers from the next shift to come to work early that day and join their team meeting whenever they can. This allows those from the later shift to learn what is happening with the day shift team, which they can then share with their own team. Some teams have their meetings begin the last 15 minutes of their shift and then continue into the first 15 minutes of the next shift so that the direct care workers of the next shift can join them for part of their meeting. Although this has the advantage of shifts learning from one another, invariably one or more people on the team cannot stay the extra 15 minutes, typically because of family commitments such as picking up a child or taking a spouse to work. Another choice of day shift teams has been to meet after serving breakfast and bathing patients but before lunch, and this has worked. Evening teams typically choose to meet after residents have gone to bed and rounds have been completed. The trainer's responsibility in this session is to provide the direct care workers with such information about the logistics of EWTs so that the team can make the best choice.

When considering the location of the team meetings, the EWTs should be assisted in deciding where they will meet each week. The teams will need a location that is private enough so that discussions are heard by no one other than the team members and the team will not be disturbed or interrupted by residents or anyone else.

The EWT members should be instructed to plan ahead on the day of their weekly team meeting. More specifically, each team member must make an effort to get her or his work completed earlier than usual on the day of the team meeting so that everyone can attend the meeting without compromising resident care. Furthermore, in the NH setting the direct care workers should be informed that the nurses will be responding to call lights while they are in their meeting. It is also important to stress that direct care worker paperwork should not be done during the team meeting.

A separate training session can be used to review the team agenda and assist the team in developing an agenda that members will be comfortable with. In this session, a sample agenda can be presented (see Exhibit 11A at the end of the chapter), and the team can be informed that it will use a different training session to examine the specific items to be covered each week.

A copy of the note sheet that teams fill out during each team meeting should be handed out to all team members for their inspection (see Exhibit 11B at the end of the chapter). Team members should observe that there is space available for all team members to sign in. This will allow managers and nurses to see who should be commended for attending the team meetings and who needs more encouragement. There is also space for one of the team members to record the minutes of the meeting, including all relevant discussions, information sharing that occurs during the meeting, recommendations being made by the team, and any questions that the team has for nurse management. On the second page of the note sheet is space for nurse management to respond to the team notes and to provide answers to questions, assuming the answers are fairly straightforward. If a question requires a complex answer, nurse management may choose to attend a portion of the team's meeting or call a separate meeting in order to provide a thorough answer.

Another issue for the team to address is who will serve as the team leader and who will take team notes. The team leader is responsible primarily for making sure everyone knows about and attends the upcoming meeting, leading the team through the agenda, and encouraging team members to share their opinions and provide their knowledge about the residents. In most cases, it is best for the team to make this decision at its first team meeting, when only the team members and facilitator are present, so that the team members will feel freer to express their opinions. In this case, the team members should be told that their first task when meeting as a team is to select a team leader, a backup team leader, and a note taker. However, it should be clarified that there are many variations to this model that the team can select, and what works best for a team seems to depend on the particular members of the team. For example, some teams may decide to rotate the team leader responsibility from week to week or month to month. In other cases, a team leader and backup are selected to serve for the first months of the team's existence. In either case, it should be clarified that the team members can vote to remove a team leader at any time that a majority of the team members think the team leader is not performing the task well (e.g., the team leader starts to boss others around or the team leader makes decisions for the team rather than facilitating team discussion and decision making).

The team note taker is responsible for taking notes during the team meeting and recording all activities unless the team members request that certain discussions not be reported or at least not be associated with particular team members. In other words, the notes are intended to be useful to managers and nurses by providing valuable information about the residents and concerns of the EWT. They should not be used to place blame on specific people unless the team specifically gives a warning to a team member who is not upholding the responsibilities of a direct care worker. It is important to clarify that the notes need not use correct spelling, grammar, or sentence structure. The only requirement is that the manager or nurse who reads the notes can understand the points being made. Here again, some teams choose to rotate note taking rather than having the same person take notes at each meeting.

Finally, this session can be used to introduce the team facilitator to the team and to clarify the facilitator's roles. The facilitator role is discussed in detail below in the section on training the facilitator. This information should be shared with the team so that all members understand their relationship to the facilitator.

SUBSEQUENT TRAINING
SESSION: THE TEAM MEETING AGENDA

A sample EWT meeting agenda should be presented to the direct care workers, and each item on the agenda should be reviewed with them so that they understand what they should spend time discussing each week. A sample meeting agenda for a day shift EWT in an NH is provided in Exhibit 11A. This sample agenda can be modified by management, nurses, and the direct care workers so that it includes all issues of importance to nurse management and the EWTs, whether in a home care, assisted living, or NH setting. A typical agenda will begin by directing the team to look for any comments or questions left in their notebook by nurse management. Such comments might be in response to the team notes from the previous week or in reference to something that has occurred during the week. If nurse management has a project or problem for the team to address that is fairly simple, this is a place where it can be left for the EWT to find and work on. If the project or problem is more complex or of extreme importance, nurse management can present the issue to the team in person during the EWT meeting and in written form.

    The agenda also typically includes time for the team members to bring up any issues, procedures, or topics that they have questions or concerns about. Some of these will be directly related to resident care. For example, when reviewing residents, a team member may have a question about the type of pureed food available for a particular resident or may express a concern that the current shower schedule is not being adhered to and needs to be revised. These issues can be discussed and where appropriate brought to the attention of nurse management. Other issues for discussion may be more directly related to workplace procedures. For example, in one case a team member expressed her frustration to the team by noting that during mealtime all the direct care workers are in the dining room except for her because she is responsible for taking trays to the immobile residents who receive meals in their rooms. Because she is the only direct care worker on the floor, she is expected to answer all the call lights during mealtime and take meal trays to resident rooms. She explained that some days it is impossible to answer all the call lights and get the meal trays to residents in a timely manner. After she presented her problem in a team meeting, the team developed new procedures for handing out meal trays so that this problem was eliminated. Team notes were used to inform nurse management of the problem and how the team planned to correct it.

    Other issues may concern staffing or interactions with nurses. For example, one of the direct care workers complained in a meeting that a particular nurse would ask her to do something when she was in the middle of assisting a resident. The team suggested that the direct care worker set up a meeting with the nurse and (1) explain to her the difficulty of receiving multiple requests when there is a time-consuming task at hand and (2) attempt to work with the nurse to find a way to revise the procedures for assigning tasks that would satisfy both of them. Eventually, in this case the team invited the nurse to one of their team meetings to inquire about the nurse's expectations of direct care workers and to share their expectations of nurses.

The agenda can include time to discuss the needs of any new residents and to acknowledge the residents who are no longer at the facility or otherwise no longer being served. Furthermore, the agenda should include time for the team members to discuss the mental or physical health of any long-term residents for whom one or more direct care workers have a growing concern. This can also be a time when direct care workers assist each other (and particularly new hires) by pointing out things that particular residents prefer or dislike and noting what works or does not work for particular residents.

The agenda can include a time to inform direct care workers of any incident reports and to discuss any future actions that should occur in response to the report. For example, a direct care worker might inform the team that she or he made an incident report after being bitten by a resident. The team would then discuss what might have caused the resident to bite and what can be done to avoid such incidents in the future.

Finally, the agenda should include a time for the direct care workers to reflect on their team work. Direct care workers can use this time to bring up any issues or concerns they have with others on their team regarding their work performance and willingness to assist others. For example, if a team member has been unwilling to assist others when called on, the team may use this time to discuss the importance of supporting one another and may even single out the negligent direct care worker, noting specific examples where help was not provided and making suggestions on how the direct care worker might perform better in the future. Of course, this must be done in a sensitive manner that emphasizes the importance of teamwork and attempts to avoid damaging morale.

SUBSEQUENT TRAINING SESSION: TEAM PROBLEM SOLVING AND DECISION MAKING

When the EWT is asked to find a solution to a workplace problem, identify an effective work procedure, or otherwise make a workplace decision, it is recommended that the direct care workers be taught to use a rational choice approach. This is a premeditated, planned approach with formal, explicit decision-making steps. To find the best solution or identify the most appropriate work procedures, prescribed steps are followed in a sequential process. Ideally, the team will have time to do the following:

1. Identify the problem to be solved or procedure to be developed.

2. Identify how the problem or procedure affects residents and staff.

3. Generate multiple alternative courses of action.

4. Carefully weigh the strengths and weaknesses of each alternative.

5. Choose the alternative that provides the most appropriate solution for solving the problem or offers the best procedure.

6. Describe the selected solution or procedure to nurse management and request feedback.

In carrying out these steps, the team members can be taught to use the form provided in Exhibit 11C at the end of the chapter. Team members should be encouraged to keep the health and satisfaction of the residents foremost in their minds when seeking possible solutions or work procedures (Steps 1 and 2). When generating possible alternatives in Step 3, the team members can be encouraged to examine how other teams or organizations address the same problem or work procedure. In some cases this can include visiting other organizations and interviewing people who have addressed the problem in the past, including other direct care workers and nurses. All ideas suggested by team members should be considered, even if they seem unrealistic. Considering all possibilities will help the team identify the best alternative.

In the process of choosing the best alternative (Steps 4 and 5) it is important to emphasize that all team members should provide input. Furthermore, the team members should be taught where varying kinds of information can be found. This might include a visit to the team from the food service and house cleaning directors. Finally, as part of the problem-solving process, it is important that the team be encouraged to select and provide a solution or procedure to nurse management in a timely fashion.

Unfortunately, it is not always possible to follow a premeditated, planned approach. In some cases, decisions must be made immediately without taking the time for the aforementioned steps. In these cases the direct care worker may be simply reacting quickly in order to take advantage of an opportunity that has presented itself, respond to an unexpected event that has occurred, or respond to task demands that require an immediate solution. This immediate decision making is unlike the rational choice method because large amounts of time are not devoted to generating alternatives, evaluating the strengths and weaknesses of each, and selecting the best one. If possible, a brief stand-up meeting with all team members present occurs and a decision is made. Procedures and solutions to problems typically are chosen quickly in order to respond to the immediate situation or to eliminate a problem quickly. Team members should be made conscious of these situations and encouraged to recognize when decisions have been made without a thorough consideration of alternatives. In such cases, the team can consider such quick decisions as temporary and then take time to identify the best alternative when time permits.

The process of decision making (as opposed to problem solving) is the process the team members will follow to select what they believe is the best alternative (Step 5 of the problem-solving process). The typical processes used are decisions by consensus or by majority vote. The process of consensus entails selecting a decision that all team members are willing to support and no team member opposes. The decision is not necessarily a unanimous choice, but it must be acceptable to all team members. All team members must have the opportunity to participate actively in the consideration and selection of the decision. Here, the "rule of thumb" procedure might be used. That is, team members use their thumbs to create three signals to show how they feel about an alternative solution. A "thumbs up" signal indicates that a team member is in favor of the solution. The "thumbs down" sign means that the member is opposed to the solution and in no way can support it. If a team member is not wild about a solution but can support it, he or she will turn the thumb sideways. If any member is "thumbs down" on a proposed solution, it may have to be modified in a way that the resister can buy in. Thus this "rule of thumb" procedure clarifies what must occur during the consensus process. Only when no team members show a "thumbs down" for a particular decision is consensus reached. In these cases all team members either support or can live with the decision.

Numerous advantages have been attributed to the consensus process. It has been described as enhancing the opportunity for innovation, creativity, and high-quality decisions because team members may spend many hours looking for an alternative that is acceptable to all. The process has been described as creating a win–win situation and enhancing trust because discussions tend to clarify and account for individual team members' reasons for their choices. Furthermore, consensus has been reported to create commitment for the decision because it is acceptable to everyone and not considered to be a bad decision by anyone (Department of Defense, 1994; Johnson & Johnson, 1994; Plunkett & Fournier, 1991).

Unfortunately, the process of consensus can also have detrimental effects. These tend to occur when a decision must be made quickly, such as in a crisis. In these cases there is typically not enough time to come to a consensus. If the team insists on obtaining a consensus, the advantages of making a quick decision may be lost, or the crisis may overwhelm the team before it has time to react. Thus using consensus as a decision-making process is advantageous to the extent that there is time available to reach a consensus, the decision is important to the team's performance, and it is important that team members be committed to the decision reached. It becomes detrimental in situations that require a quick decision.

The process of majority rule entails taking a vote of team members to determine which of several decisions will be selected by the team. The decision receiving a majority of the votes is the one selected. Typically, the process is to discuss an issue until at least 51% of the members agree on a decision.

The use of majority rule is particularly advantageous for teams when sufficient time is lacking for decision by consensus or when the decision is not so important that the time-consuming consensus process is needed. In other words, some decisions simply do not warrant the time, effort, and energy that consensus entails. Majority rule also becomes an advantage when a decision cannot be reached by consensus and may be the best process when commitment by all team members is not necessary for implementing the decision.

When majority rule is used, it is important that all team members feel that they have had an opportunity to express their view, that their view was seriously considered, and that all team members feel that the decision made is not for an individual's personal gain or advantage. The use of majority rule appears to be particularly detrimental when commitment to the decision is needed by all team members in order for it to be implemented. Majority rule can result in some team members feeling as if they are the winners while others feel as if they are the losers. In these cases the "losers" can be expected to show little commitment to carrying out the majority decision. The use of majority rule can also be detrimental when the decision is personally important to the team members, such as establishing who will serve which residents. Those in the minority may take the vote personally and feel that others on the team are getting back at them for earlier disagreements. Such problems, stemming from the majority rule process, have been found to result in difficulty implementing the decisions made by the EWT at best and to resentment, distrust, conflict, and dissolution of the team at worst. Furthermore, the majority rule process can result in lower-quality decisions. In these cases inadequate time is devoted to reviewing the pros and cons of alternative choices before a vote is taken.

Thus the trainer should help each team recognize when consensus is the best decision-making process and when it is best to use majority rule. The team should be encouraged to use majority rule when there is need to make a quick decision, when the decision is not particularly important to the team members, or when the team is having difficulty making the decision by consensus. Consensus should be sought when the solution selected will have large effects on the residents, staff, or organization (i.e., it is an important decision), when the decision is important to all the team members, or when the solution selected will require a high level of commitment from all team members to be implemented successfully.

SUBSEQUENT TRAINING SESSION: INTERPERSONAL PROCESSES

All direct care workers need good or at least adequate interpersonal skills in order to work effectively with coworkers, nurses, managers, and residents. These skills typically include communicating, listening with empathy, questioning, clarifying and confirming, resolving conflict, and working collaboratively. These skills become particularly important when direct care workers work in EWTs where opposing ideas are periodically considered by the team members and attempts are made to reach a consensus. Teaching interpersonal skills is not an easy task. The trainer may choose to look for a packaged training program designed to teach interpersonal skills or turn to an experienced consultant. If a packaged interpersonal training program is chosen, it must include a focus on communication and cooperative conflict.

EWT members will need good communication skills, particularly when participating in their team meetings. It is important that team members be instructed to

- Present information to each other in a clear manner.

- Listen closely to what each team member says.

- Understand each other without misinterpreting what is being said.

- Be sensitive to one another's feelings.

- Focus on team issues, not personalities.

One means of emphasizing the importance of communication is through examples from the long-term care setting of good and poor communication. In our experience, one clear example from an NH was the lack of communication between two team members who had been close friends. This friendship came to an end when one of the team members believed that the other had spoken with their supervisor and wrongly accused her of poor performance. As a result, these two direct care workers never spoke to one another and had not assisted one another with work activities for weeks. This included not helping one another with lifting heavy patients, even when the alternative was lifting a patient single-handedly. This lack of communication and teamwork negatively affected their ability to do a good job and could have easily resulted in one or both of the direct care workers getting injured as they attempted to lift heavy patients. The lack of communication was overcome when an EWT was created on their floor. In the very first meeting, one of the two direct care workers raised the issue of trust. In the ensuing discussion, the one direct care worker learned that the other had not reported her to their supervisor as first believed. This resulted in the two apologizing. As a result, the barriers to communication between them were removed, and they began helping one another, sharing information, and enjoying their jobs more.

One means of teaching good communication skills is to create one or more role-playing situations. For example, the team members might be given a fictitious problem to solve with each team member, given facts to share and a description of the type of person they are to represent (e.g., confrontational, friendly, bossy, low self-esteem). One team member should also be assigned the team leader role. The team members can then practice sharing information, listening, providing and receiving feedback, solving problems, and dealing with conflict. The trainer can assist them in seeing how attitudes can get in the way of good communication and can help the team to see how the team leader needs to act as a facilitator of discussion and not a new supervisor for the direct care workers.

Conflict between team members is a natural occurrence that can lead to either problems and dysfunctional behavior or to beneficial behavior. *Beneficial or cooperative conflict* refers to situations in which two or more team members have opposing ideas and views but are motivated to explore and understand the views and interests of others. Typically each person is willing to accept that his or her own perspective has shortcomings, appreciates and respects the goals of the other, tries to integrate other ideas with his or her own, and strives to develop mutually satisfactory decisions based on everyone's input. The use of cooperative conflict results in strengthened relationships and confidence that conflicts can be resolved in the future.

On the other hand, dysfunctional or competitive conflict exists when people choose to defend their own positions vigorously and attempt to win over others. Team members try to understand the other's view only to find weaknesses, not to modify their own perspective. In this way, conflict results in a failure to reach an agreement, and in its place a solution may be imposed by the more powerful team members. The use of competitive conflict results in weakened relationships and a lack of confidence that conflicts can be resolved in the future. Furthermore, because the solutions reached are not supported or at least accepted by everyone on the team, it is possible that some team members may attempt to sabotage the success of the team. These important distinctions between cooperative conflict and competitive conflict should be pointed out to the team members.

Team members should also become aware of the factors that can facilitate cooperative conflict. These include the following:

- *Give teammates a chance to say what they think.* Be sure the other direct care workers are given a chance to express their ideas about whatever the team is considering. Let everyone have a chance to say what they are thinking. For those who have not volunteered their thoughts on the issue, it would be good to give them a chance to speak up by asking them whether they have any thoughts they would like to share.

- *Listen.* When a team member is sharing her thoughts, all other direct care workers should be carefully listening to her and trying to understand why she feels and thinks the way she does. Team members should ask her questions where needed to be sure her viewpoint is understood and the facts she is using to come to her conclusions are known.

- Each team member should *share her or his thoughts* on the issue of concern. This should include not only one's opinion but also the information and knowledge used to reach the opinion.

- Remember that *no idea is a bad idea*. A teammate should never be told that her or his idea is a stupid one. When this happens, people will stop sharing their thoughts. Simply ask the person to explain further. If the idea is not a good one, that is okay because the team needs to consider many ideas in order to identify the best one.

SUBSEQUENT TRAINING SESSIONS: SCENARIOS, "PLAY BALL," AND EFFECTIVE TEAMS

As with the managers and nurses described in Chapter 10, the direct care workers can be provided subsequent training that includes a review of scenarios (see Chapter 10, Exhibit 10A) and the "play ball" technique so that the team members see how managers, nurses, and EWTs are to work together in reaching solutions to problems and designing programs. A review of the requirements for effective teams (see Chapter 10) will likewise help the direct care workers understand their new responsibilities, as will a discussion of the criteria for obtaining a team excellence award (see Chapter 10, Exhibit 10B).

SUBSEQUENT TRAINING SESSION: AN OVERVIEW OF THE TRAINING THAT MANAGEMENT AND NURSES, TEAM FACILITATORS, TEAM LEADERS, AND HUMAN RESOURCE STAFF ARE RECEIVING

The direct care workers should be given an overview of the training that other employees are receiving. This will teach them what is expected of these other employees and what the other employees will expect of them.

Training Team Facilitators

This training should be targeted to employees who will be facilitating the EWTs. When a team facilitator is being selected, the following characteristics should be considered:

- A team facilitator should be a person not supervising the direct care workers. Otherwise, the team members will not feel free to say what they think during team meetings and are likely to be concerned that if they say the "wrong" thing, the facilitator–supervisor could hold it against them later, resulting in a poor evaluation, lower wages, and possibly loss of their job.

- A team facilitator should be someone respected, trusted, and liked by the direct care workers. The facilitator will be constantly evaluating the activities and behaviors of the direct care workers and identifying those that are inconsistent with a team approach. The facilitator will also be correcting direct care workers as needed, such as when one team member says things in a team meeting that are insensitive to another. The team members are more likely to listen and change their behavior if the constructive criticism comes from someone they respect, trust, and like.

- A team facilitator should be someone who is respected by management and nurses. The facilitator will at times be a mediator between the team and nurse management. To be effective, the facilitator will need the respect of the managers and nurses.

- A team facilitator should be someone who has strong interpersonal skills that can be taught to the direct care workers. Without strong interpersonal skills, it may be difficult for the team facilitator to recognize when these skills are lacking in others. Furthermore, it takes strong interpersonal skills to be able to effectively correct inappropriate behaviors of others.

In some cases, the trainer may be able to serve as a team's facilitator. Other people who might be suitable are those who have worked as direct care workers in the past but have been promoted to other positions, such as a medical aide or perhaps a licensed practical nurse (2-year post–high school education). In some cases, a person from outside the organization can serve as a team facilitator if the person has the necessary skills, is not believed to be working for management, and has the respect of the direct care workers.

The team facilitator will be responsible for the following (see Exhibit 11D):

- Helping the team leader gather the direct care workers together each week on their selected meeting day and time.

- Attending the team meetings each week and assisting the team leader in making sure that all team members sign in at the beginning of the meeting, review and stay focused on the agenda items and other issues to be discussed, and have an opportunity to give input. Furthermore, the facilitator should help the team leader make sure that someone on the team takes notes and that the notes are provided to nurse management each week. As the direct care workers become more proficient in their team meetings, the team facilitator should begin skipping some of the weekly meetings. As time moves on and the team becomes more adept, the team facilitator will attend fewer and fewer meetings.

- Acting as a sounding board for the team members by helping them to see when they have been insensitive to one another or have otherwise displayed poor interpersonal skills (e.g., dominating conversations, ignoring the input of others, making fun of others' ideas). For some problems (e.g., making fun of oth-

---

EXHIBIT 11D.
Responsibilities of the Team Facilitator

For a newly developing team to be most effective, it needs a facilitator at the team's weekly meetings. Each facilitator should do the following:

- *Make sure that the team meets each week.* If the direct care workers are coming to the meetings late, the facilitator and team leader can request that the director of nursing meet with the team to emphasize the importance of the weekly meetings.

- *Make sure that the team reviews the weekly agenda (and each item on it).* This will include reading what the nurse management has left for the team to discuss, reviewing resident needs, and considering any issues brought up by team members. If the direct care workers are not getting or staying focused on the agenda items, the facilitator will need to encourage this. For example, one of the agenda items is, "Have you had any positive experiences you would like to share?" If there is no response, the facilitator might say something like, "Are you sure there isn't something or someone positive that you can report? Were there any nurses who were helpful this past week?"

- *Make sure that someone on the team takes notes of what was discussed during the meeting.* The facilitator may need to remind the note taker to take notes in cases where the note taker has forgotten to record something of importance that was discussed.

- *Make sure that nurse management reads and responds to the direct care workers' notes.* Otherwise the direct care workers will feel as if they are wasting their time.

- *Be neutral and nonthreatening to the direct care workers.*

- *Assist the team as needed through the problem-solving process.*

- *Attempt to assist the direct care workers with their interpersonal skills while being respectful and nonthreatening.* It is useful in the beginning for the team to determine what behaviors are not acceptable, such as chatting, participating in non–work-related discussions, or personally attacking a member who has made a suggestion. It is also important for team members to respect team members from different ethnic backgrounds.

- *Help the direct care workers use cooperative conflict and discourage competitive conflict.*

- *Provide hands-on assistance in the beginning* but be less involved as the team matures by participating less in team meetings and eventually attending fewer and fewer meetings.

ers) the facilitator may choose to address the problem to the team as a whole. For other problems (e.g., dominating a discussion) the facilitator may meet privately with particular team members to discuss the importance of allowing everyone time to speak. In either case, it is helpful when the facilitator can provide examples of desirable behavior.

- Helping the direct care workers to work through the problem-solving process as they seek solutions to problems or develop new work procedures. The facilitator should not provide substantive input regarding solutions to problems or effective work procedures; that is the role of the EWT. The facilitator should help the direct care workers follow the steps in the problem-solving process so that the team can identify the best possible solution or work procedure.

- Making sure that nurse management is responding each week to the notes left by the teams.

- Acting as a mediator between the team and nurse management when there are apparent misunderstandings.

- Encouraging managers and nurses to empower the EWTs and pointing out situations that appear ideal for this (e.g., nurse management is developing a new procedure for handing out meal trays and is encouraged by the team facilitator to turn this responsibility over to the team or at least allow them to provide input).

Team facilitators should begin their training by attending all management and direct care worker training sessions. Through these, the facilitator will gain an understanding of the goals of the teams and how they are to achieve their goals and will learn the roles and responsibilities of management and nurses as they relate to the EWTs. Next, the facilitators should be taught their own responsibilities, as described earlier. This training can be supplemented by visiting with and learning from others who have already worked as team facilitators and by attending training sessions for team facilitators provided at conferences or by private consultants (e.g., the Center for Collaborative Organizations at the University of North Texas).

Training Team Leaders

The team leader of an EWT should be one of the team's members who is selected by the team (Exhibit 11E). Likewise, the team members should select a second person who will fill in during a team leader's absence. The team members should be taught the responsibilities of the team leader during their orientation and training and be aware that the team will be responsible for selecting someone to fill this role. This will give them time to discuss and consider possible team leaders and to learn which direct care workers are willing to take on this responsibility. Team leaders typically are identified during the first team meeting. In some cases, several people may be willing to take on this responsibility, with team members willing to support either. In these cases, the team may choose to have people rotate the team leader position from week to week, have one person serve as team leader for a given period of weeks and then the other, or have co–team leaders facilitate each team meeting. This latter solution has been found to be particularly effective where the two co-leaders highly respect one another.

It will be beneficial to provide the team leader with training that reviews the responsibilities of the team leader and provides instruction on how to facilitate meetings and encourage good interpersonal skills among team members. Unfortunately, if this training is limited to only the one direct care worker who will be serving as the team leader, then some of the other direct care workers are likely to develop the mistaken belief that the team leader is receiving special treatment from management. Furthermore, the team leader may get this feeling also and begin to take on a more authoritative role during the team meetings. Consequently, it is best if the training of the team leader is not limited to those who will be taking on this responsibility. Instead, all team members should receive the team leader training. This has multiple benefits that include allowing all team members to understand the responsibilities of the team leader, avoiding a misunderstanding of the team leader's relationship with management, and providing interpersonal skill training to all team members.

The primary responsibilities of the team leader include the following:

- Reminding the team members of their upcoming weekly team meeting and, on the day of the meeting, encouraging them to get their work completed in a timely way so they can attend the meeting without leaving work undone.

- Making sure that the location for the team meeting is available, that the team members sign in as they arrive for the meeting, and that the note taker has retrieved the team's notebook.

EXHIBIT 11E.
The Team Leader

- *What is a team leader?* A team leader is a member of the team who is willing to lead the team through the agenda during weekly meetings and to facilitate short stand-up meetings when needed. A team leader is not a supervisor of other direct care workers.

- *Who can be a team leader?* Any team member who has the interest to serve in this capacity, has the support of her or his teammates, and can be counted on to hold team meetings on time, keep the team focused on the team agenda, and encourage involvement of all team members.

- *Who can select a team leader?* Team members can select their own team leader. Team members know their own teammates' abilities and skills better than anyone else and know who they are likely to feel comfortable with to lead their team meetings. In some cases, nurse management may initially appoint a team leader with the understanding that team members will select their own leader later.

- Leading the team through the meeting agenda (Exhibit 11A) and encouraging discussion and input from all team members. This includes asking for opinions from team members who do not naturally speak up and sensitively asking those who tend to dominate discussions to give others an opportunity to share their thoughts and relevant information. It also includes making sure that the team members are not doing something else while attending the team meeting, such as completing resident charts.

- Keeping the team focused on the agenda items or other issues of concern to the team. Discussions can sometimes get off track, or at times a single person can begin to dominate a discussion or keep the team focused on an issue of personal concern. For example, we observed this occurring just before a team member quit, with the team member wanting to spend the majority of each team meeting on the reasons why he was going to quit. It is the responsibility of the team leader to prevent a team member from dominating the discussion or the topic under discussion. Likewise, the team leader should be sure that she is not dominating the discussions herself.

- Displaying and encouraging good interpersonal skills. Although discussions can get heated at times, with varying opinions being expressed, there should be no name calling or other disrespecting of others. The team leader is responsible for maintaining civil behavior between team members as cooperative conflict occurs. Likewise, the team leader should exemplify and encourage clear communication and listening.

- Making sure that the team's notebook is made available to nurse management after the team meeting.

As noted earlier, team leader training should be provided to all team members. The team trainer can review for them the team leader's responsibilities. Interpersonal skill training can be provided by the trainer, by a private consultant, or through the use of packaged training programs. This should include skill development in communication, listening, cooperative conflict, compromising, being flexible, and being respectful. Role playing can be an effective part of this training, with some team members displaying disrespectful behavior and others practicing how to defuse such situations and encourage good interpersonal skills.

Sample Agenda for Empowered Work Team Meetings: Day Shift

1. Please read our notes from last week and the responses from the nurse staff. Do we want to make any additional comments? Are there any issues the nurses want us to discuss or responses we want to make?

2. Are there any issues or procedures related to our work that you would like to discuss today? (Give people a minute to think.)

3. Is there anyone here who worked the night shift? If so, could you give us an update?

4. Do we have any new residents? Can someone give us an update on her or him?

5. Has anyone completed an incident report recently? If so, please tell us what happened.

6. Have any of the residents on your hall developed a skin problem or stopped eating? What are you doing to help them with these problems? Any recommendations?

7. Have any residents displayed new behavioral problems? What are you doing, if anything, to address these problems?

8. Have you had any positive experiences that you would like to share?

9. Have you had any problems that you would like to share? Maybe someone on the team will have a suggestion for what to do.

10. Is there anything that has happened recently and you do not understand why it happened?

11. Are there any new members on our team? If so, do they have any questions about the work or residents?

12. How are we doing in terms of teamwork? Anything else?

13. Please read back our notes for today.

14. Okay, our meeting is adjourned.

Empowered Work Team Meeting Notes

Date: _____

	Name	Time		Name	Time
1.			6.		
2.			7.		
3.			8.		
4.			9.		
5.			10.		

Notes: _____

_____

_____

_____

_____

_____

_____

_____

_____

_____

_____

_____

_____

_____

_____

_____

Recorded by: _____

(continued)

EWT Meeting Notes *(continued):* Date: _____

Notes (*continued*):

_____

_____

_____

_____

_____

_____

_____

_____

Response from Nurse Management:

_____

_____

_____

_____

_____

_____

_____

_____

_____

_____

_____

Recorded by: _____

Empowered Work Teams in Long-Term Care. © 2008 Health Professions Press. All rights reserved.

Steps for Finding a Solution to a Current Problem

Date: _____

1. Describe an issue, problem, or question related to our work.

   _____

   _____

   _____

   _____

2. How does it affect the residents and staff?

   _____

   _____

   _____

   _____

3. List at least two possible solutions and the strengths and weaknesses of each (use next page if needed).

   _____

   _____

   _____

   _____

4. Discuss each possible solution and be sure to consider the following:

   a. What must be done to accomplish the solution.

   b. What problems might be caused by the solution? For example,

   • How does the solution affect the residents?
   • Are the necessary resources, such as money and equipment, available?
   • Does the solution ignore any laws or company policies?

5. After discussing each of the possible solutions, choose the best one.

6. Provide the team's choice to the nursing supervisors, along with this worksheet, and ask for feedback.

CHAPTER 12

Maintaining Effective Teams in Long-Term Care
What Must Go Right and What Can Go Wrong

Empowered work teams (EWTs) have been found to have many positive effects, including improved resident care, work processes, and work attitudes as well as reduced turnover. However, if managers, nurses, and direct care workers are not performing their responsibilities, as described in previous chapters, these effects will not be realized. The key to success is getting the teams started correctly and then maintaining the same procedures and behaviors over time. Described in this chapter are some of the practices that can help or hinder the teams as they work to enhance resident health and maintain positive employee attitudes.

MANAGERS MUST KEEP THE TEAM INVOLVED

A problem typically found among the EWTs in the authors' study is the lack of attention by managers and nurses (henceforth called managers) responsible for communicating and working with the team. These managers have two primary responsibilities. The first is to respond to any comments or questions that the team presents to them through their weekly notebook or verbal questioning. The second is to provide the team with decision-making opportunities. With regard to responding to comments or questions, it is important that the team's manager always respond to the comments in the team's notebook each week. The direct care workers are making an effort to meet, discuss the health of the residents they serve, and consider how work procedures can be improved to better serve the residents. When the team's managers neglect to read the team's notes and to seriously consider their recommendations, the team becomes demoralized, and its effectiveness decreases.

The managers should also routinely give the EWT a decision-making opportunity that allows the direct care workers to participate in workplace changes that affect them. For example, at one extreme this can include important decisions such as developing weekly procedures for ensuring that all residents are bathed regularly or deciding whether to hire a prospective applicant. At the other extreme, the decision-making opportunity might be less dramatic, such as asking the team to develop a list of resident preferences and then keeping the list at the front desk or attaching them to the backs of the residents' closet doors so that new or temporary direct care workers can easily learn the individual preferences of the residents being served. Whether they are "important" decisions or less so, the team needs regular opportunities to be involved in making decisions. Such involvement will maintain the direct care workers' enthusiasm for the team. And, just as importantly, it will take advantage of the knowledge that the direct care workers have to offer.

PREVENT A SINGLE TEAM MEMBER FROM DOMINATING TEAM MEETINGS

EWTs are most successful when all the team members participate during team meetings, including reviewing resident health and making decisions about the work. Such involvement takes advantage of all the knowledge available among the direct care workers and heightens their feelings of self-worth and job satisfaction. Unfortunately, at times a single team member may attempt to dominate the team meetings, usually by controlling what is discussed or not giving others much opportunity to speak. There are at least two reasons why this occurs. In one case, the team member is dissatisfied with the job or with some particular aspect of the job and insists that the team stay focused on her or his dissatisfactions. In other cases the team member believes she is the most knowledgeable person on the team and so knows best what the team should discuss.

In the case of a dissatisfied team member, the person dominates team meetings by insisting on discussing a particular topic even after the team has thoroughly discussed the topic and the rest of the team is ready to move on to other topics. For example, in one case a direct care worker appeared to be burned out from the job and as a result wanted to spend the whole team meeting complaining about how there was not enough time to get the work done and spend time with the residents. In another case the team member wanted to spend the whole team meeting complaining about the poor treatment she was receiving from a particular nurse. The appropriate response from the rest of the team is to pay close attention to the complaining person and to provide suggestions on how she can resolve the issues, whether it is talking with the director of nursing about the work procedures or taking a troublesome nurse aside to discuss the issues of concern. Typically, providing suggestions to the troubled team member can take a majority of a team's weekly meeting time. However, this is time well spent if the dominating team member listens to the team's suggestions, carries them out, and is subsequently able to resolve the issue of concern. The dominating team member becomes a problem for the team when the team meets the next week and the same team member begins to again dominate the meeting time by complaining about the same problems. When they ask whether she has attempted to implement any of the suggestions offered the previous week by the team (e.g., "Take the nurse aside and tell her how you feel"), the team learns that she has not. At this point, the dominating behavior must not be allowed to continue because it prevents the team from addressing other issues, and the constant complaining creates a negative feeling within the team.

A team member who dominates discussions because he believes he has more experience and knowledge than the others on the team will dominate the meeting by presenting what he believes is the right decision, going into detail about why his decision is the best one and quickly pointing out flaws in any opposing solutions suggested by others. Typically, other team members are not given the same amount of time to describe their potential solution before being shown why their suggestion is inferior. This results in team members not wanting to make suggestions and losing interest in the team discussions altogether. This dominating behavior appears to be most common among team leaders because they are in a position to present their ideas first and to cut off the discussion of others. Furthermore, team members typically feel obligated to defer to the dominating team member because of her or his extensive knowledge.

The best solution for overcoming a dominating team member is for one or more other team members to request assistance from the team facilitator. A person from outside the team often is viewed as more objective and can help the dominating person recognize the problem. Furthermore, the team facilitator can assist the dominating person in receiving training that is designed to help the person see how he or she is dominating discussions and what she or he can do to prevent it.

TEAM LEADERS MUST ENCOURAGE PARTICIPATION

It has been shown in earlier chapters that team member participation in decision making can result in better decisions, improved work attitudes, and more willingness to carry out the decisions made. However, some team members are introverted by nature and consequently are not particularly comfortable sharing their ideas, even when their ideas are excellent ones. Other team members may be more extroverted but lack confidence when it comes to participating in decision making and subsequently have little to say when the time comes. In either case, it is imperative that the team leader encourage all team members to contribute to team discussions. One method for doing this is to ask particularly quiet people for their opinions during the team meeting. Another is to routinely go around the table from person to person, asking each to share her or his thoughts on the problem being addressed by the team. During this exercise, the team leader might probe for more information from the team members who are shy or lack the confidence to describe in detail what they are thinking. What will especially influence participation of these and other team members is positive feedback when someone shares an idea. Participants should feel that they will be respected for anything that they share and that they will not be criticized or ridiculed even when others disagree with them.

NURSES AND MANAGERS MUST SUPPORT THE TEAM

EWTs cannot be successful on their own; they need to be supported by both nurses and managers. This includes receiving all relevant information related to a decision and being provided enough time to consider alternative choices before revising a work process. The team will not be successful if managers have not taken the time to consider what information the direct care workers will need and provide this information to them. Furthermore, team members should feel that they can go to managers and nurses for information or invite a manager or nurse to their team meeting so they can ask questions related to the issue they are addressing.

Support from managers and nurses also means covering for the direct care workers for 30 minutes or so while they hold their weekly team meeting. The team will not be successful if team members must routinely leave their meeting to answer call lights or are routinely pulled out of the meeting by a nurse for other reasons. Undoubtedly there are times when a direct care worker must be pulled away to help address an immediate problem. However, this should be the exception rather than the norm.

Finally, the team members need encouragement from their supervisors and others so that they feel that their suggestions will be respected and taken seriously. The team needs to hear that they are capable of making good decisions, that they have the complete support of management and nurses, and that any questions or requests they have will be taken seriously and answered promptly. This does not mean that whatever the team wants will be granted. But it does mean that the "play ball" process will be taken seriously and that management and nurse support will go beyond verbal encouragement to include specific actions that will ensure that the EWT is involved in decision making.

KEEPING THE EWTS EXCITING

Empowering direct care workers can have very positive effects on job attitudes and can result in the direct care workers enthusiastically implementing the decisions made rather than doing so halfheartedly. It is the EWT that provides an effective means of empowering the direct care workers. However, over time the EWTs, managers, and nurses can develop habits and procedures that appear to lessen direct care worker empowerment and thus the excitement of participating in decision making. For example, in some cases the EWT meetings become very routine, with the same few team members doing all the participating in the decisions made. In other cases, the team may have strayed away from the meeting agenda so that they are no longer seeking to participate or make decisions related to their work. Here, the direct care workers find it is easier to go along with what one is told than it is to collect facts about an issue, weigh varying alternatives, and then make a recommendation that may not be accepted immediately or that might be substantially modified. In still other cases, the managers and nurses provide fewer and fewer opportunities for the EWT to participate in decision making. In these cases, the managers and nurses find it easier to make their own decision rather than describe the issue to a whole team of direct care workers, provide them with information related to the issue, "play ball" with them, and end up compromising their own views in order to account for those of the direct care workers. When the team is going through one of these scenarios, it will need assistance to get back on track so that all the team members are participating in decision making and the excitement that comes with such participation is rekindled.

One method of accomplishing this is to have the team facilitator visit one or more team meetings. The facilitator can help the team get back on track by encouraging the team to identify workplace issues that the direct care workers believe could be improved, by making sure that none of the team members, including the team leader, is dominating discussions, by making sure that all team members are participating, and by mediating any conflicts that are preventing the team meetings from being productive. Furthermore, the team facilitator may want to have the team reflect on its development and progress. For example, in one case where the team members were losing interest in the EWT, the facilitator asked the direct care workers to list the reasons why they used to look forward to participating in team meetings, why they are less interested now, and what needs to be changed so that the team meetings would become more worthwhile. In this particular case, the team members developed a list of reasons why the EWT was worthwhile to them, including learning about new changes in the workplace, obtaining clarification and reducing misunderstandings about new changes, having a means of getting the attention of management and nurses regarding issues or problems important to the direct care workers, having a stronger voice when sharing opinions than a single person would have, hands-on teaching for newer workers, maintaining friendships within and across shifts, and obtaining the opinions of other direct care workers regarding one's ideas. The facilitator was able to use this information to identify areas for improvement, such as having the managers and nurses take more time to involve the EWT in the development of the workplace changes taking place. This brought a renewed excitement to the team.

Another method is for management and nurses to build into their work routines time to identify important issues for the EWT to address. This might be a work process issue or an anticipated decision that management or a nurse will need to make. Again, the key is to present the issue to the team, including all relevant background information, allowing the team time to consider alternatives, seriously considering the suggestions offered by the team, and after "playing ball" implementing the resulting work process or decision collectively reached.

Still another method includes having the team invite managers and nurses to team meetings, with a different manager or nurse attending a portion of the meeting each week. Those invited could range from the organization's administrator or the director of food service to nurses working the same shift as the team. The team can use these meeting times to ask the invited guest how she or he perceives the team, what she or he sees as the team's responsibilities, what is perceived to be good about the team, and in what ways the team could improve. This can be particularly valuable if a particular nurse or manager is not working well with the EWTs. Such a meeting can allow for a frank discussion of expectations from both the nurse and the EWT, a look at where there are differences of opinion, and an attempt to identify common ground where all can come to an agreement about the work and the nurse–EWT relationship.

Still another strategy for increasing team excitement is to implement a team award that recognizes a team for its accomplishments (see Chapter 10). If multiple

EWTs exist in the organization, then a monthly award might be offered. As part of establishing award criteria, the team can be given an opportunity to outline what must be accomplished in order for the award to be received. This could include criteria such as number of absences among the team members, resident satisfaction with the direct care workers, or helpful recommendations provided to management and nurses. Awards can range from monetary gifts to certificates of accomplishment. Of course, monetary gifts and the like are the most preferred. As part of this award program, the team can be asked to keep track of its performance as it relates to the team award and, when the team members feel they have accomplished the award criteria, can petition management to consider them for the award.

Summary and Conclusions

Both quantitative and qualitative research have clearly shown that empowering nonmanagement employees, such as direct-care workers (DCW), can have a variety of important and very positive effects for an organization as well as for its nonmanagement employees. Feelings of empowerment can increase commitment to an organization as well as job satisfaction and self-esteem. Similarly, improved job performance, enhanced communication, and reduced burnout and turnover can result from high levels of empowerment. So the question becomes: How can feelings of empowerment be created among nonmanagement employees so that these many positive outcomes can be realized?

One answer is empowered work teams (EWT). To establish EWTs effectively, the direct-care workers must learn to communicate with each other as well as with management in a professional manner. Management must constantly work to involve the EWTs in the decision-making process and to routinely give them opportunities to make decisions about their work. Further, team practices must be constantly monitored by management and team members in order to recognize when the team is developing bad habits and to help the team get back on track. Most important, all team members should be involved in the decision-making process, all information needed to make good decisions should be provided to the team, and no one or two team members should dominate team discussions and decision-making. As shown in Section II, the results can be astounding.

EWTs can provide not only high employee empowerment and its accompanying benefits, but also an enriched environment where employees learn from one another. This has been extremely valuable in the case of certified nursing assistants (CNAs) in nursing homes. The EWTs provided CNAs time to discuss among themselves their work and their residents. CNAs learned from one another how to more effectively get their jobs done and in a timely manner, such as by getting residents up and ready for breakfast in the morning and by helping them to the toilet before bed. Further, the CNAs learned from one another the likes and dislikes of the residents, which resulted in happier, more satisfied residents. It is reasonable to suspect that such information sharing among CNAs resulted in fewer nursing home deficiencies.

Almost all recent initiatives in long-term care have encouraged more empowerment of DCWs. Unfortunately, most of these initiatives provide no clear directions on how to make this happen. This book helps to fill that gap in the knowledge base. As the empowerment of DCWs grows in long-term care and becomes more routine, the day-to-day care of residents will improve as will the attitudes of the direct care workers.

Appendix: Steps for Implementing Empowered Work Teams in Long-Term Care

The steps for implementing empowered work teams (EWTs) in long-term care (LTC) were developed from the experiences of implementing EWTs in six nursing homes (NHs). As we moved from one NH to the next we evaluated our success at each point, identified areas that could be improved, modified our steps accordingly, and then proceeded to implement teams in the next NH. Although the following steps seem very prescriptive, it should be noted that the implementation procedures used will vary from one NH to the next depending on factors such as the culture of the NH and the preferences of the managers, nurses, and direct care workers.

1. *Select someone to provide an initial orientation to staff.* The person providing the orientation should be an in-house employee who has gained knowledge of EWTs through study, conferences and workshops, and speaking and visiting with others who are using EWTs. Through these, the in-house trainer should gain a clear understanding of the purposes of the EWTs, their activities, and how they relate to management. An external consultant may also be used to teach and assist the in-house trainer. Chapter 9 provides more details.

2. *Introduce the concept of EWTs to managers and nurses.* The purpose is to provide an understanding of the goals of EWTs, how they function, how they interact with managers and nurses, and their benefits and costs. Those receiving this orientation should include the administrator, director of nursing (DON), assistant administrator and assistant DON, and nurses. Other personnel might include the organization's social worker, financial officer, human resource (HR) or personnel director, department heads, and any others in key management positions (Exhibit 9A provides orientation materials).

3. *Question the managers and nurses before deciding whether to implement EWTs.* Once managers and nurses have an understanding of EWTs, they will be in a position to provide their opinion as to whether EWTs would be successful. More specifically, they should be asked anonymously whether they believe EWTs could be successful and why or why not. Other managers, such as department heads and the HR director, can be surveyed as well (see Exhibit 9C for a brief questionnaire). Anonymity should be used to avoid receiving answers that reflect what the administrator wants rather than what the managers and nurses actually desire or believe will work.

Experience has shown that EWTs will not be successful unless management and nurses are in support of them. Managing EWTs requires that managers work with the teams, provide them with relevant information, and at times allow the teams to try things that a manager or nurse would not consider. Most importantly, managers must take time to work with the teams. Nothing was found more frustrating to team members than to work hard on developing a solution or revising a procedure and then receiving a late or no response from managers and nurses. Team members are soon heard saying, "Why work on this if it doesn't matter what we come up with anyway?" Experience with implementing EWTs suggests that it would not be fruitful to go beyond this point unless the managers and nurses believe EWTs are worth the effort.

4. *Introduce the concept of EWTs to the direct care workers and get their input.* It is not recommended to introduce the idea of EWTs to the direct care workers unless the managers and nurses are in favor of implementing them. If the direct care workers are introduced to the idea of participating in decisions and then later told that they will not have this responsibility, many of them are likely to feel disappointed and even angry. If managers and nurses are in favor of the EWTs, then the next step is to introduce the idea to the direct care workers and obtain their opinion about their desirability and potential for success. Their orientation should be similar to that provided to managers and nurses. Experience shows that most direct care workers would like to have the added responsibilities associated with EWTs, although not all would. Some direct care workers fear that they lack the skills and knowledge to carry out the new responsibilities successfully and, as a result, could lose their job if the EWTs are implemented. Others may not believe that EWTs will work because the managers and nurses involved would not allow them to be successful. However, experience shows that most direct care workers welcome the opportunity to contribute their knowledge to the decision-making process and to the development of work procedures and so are in favor of implementing EWTs. Of course, if the direct care workers as a whole are not in favor of EWTs, then they should not be implemented, and no further steps should be taken.

5. *Select and educate the EWT trainers.* Those who provided the orientation to the managers, nurses, and direct care workers are the most likely candidates to also provide the in-depth training that will be needed. This will include training sessions to detail the EWT goals and the responsibilities and activities of the EWTs as well as those of the managers, nurses, team facilitators, team leaders, and HR director. The trainers will need more knowledge than what was needed to provide the initial orientations and so should devote extensive time to studying about EWTs, attending conferences and workshops related to them, and visiting organizations that use them. The organization may also choose to involve an outside consultant who can provide guidance and assist the in-house trainers. See Chapters 9 and 10 for more details.

6. *Provide in-depth training to managers, nurses, direct care workers, team facilitators, team leaders, and HR directors.* Once it is determined that EWTs will be implemented within the organization and in-house trainers are prepared, extensive

training should be provided. The purpose of the training is to teach those being trained to understand their roles and responsibilities, as well as those of others involved in empowering the direct care workers. For all those being trained, this includes the goals of EWTs, the positive and negative effects that can occur, the roles of the team leader and team facilitator, the ways in which management should interact with the teams, the importance of allowing the teams time to develop solutions, and the benefits of allowing teams to carry out their decisions even when their decisions do not appear to be the best available (as long as their solution has no serious detrimental effects on the residents). Chapter 10 details useful information that can be taught.

It should be noted that the training should occur as close to the actual team implementation date as possible. Otherwise, when the teams finally are implemented, it will be more difficult for managers and nurses to remember to empower them, and the direct care workers will become frustrated waiting for the opportunity to participate in decision making. Because no more than a few EWTs should be implemented at one time, this means that not all the direct care workers will receive the in-depth training at the same time. Only the first teams to be implemented should receive the in-depth training at first, with additional teams receiving in-depth training only after the first teams are functioning well.

7. *Determine the logistics for the EWTs, including the number of teams, who will be on each, and when and where they will meet.* During training, the managers should decide how many teams will be established and who should be on each. Typically, teams are established based on the areas that they serve and the shift that they work. For example, an assisted living facility might have two teams, one that serves the residents during the day shift and the other that serves the residents during the evening shift. The facility might have a third team that serves the residents on the weekend if there is a permanent weekend direct care staff. It has been found that night teams usually are not viable unless they have at least five direct care workers who work the night shift regularly. It should be noted that the night shift direct care workers were found to greatly appreciate being included in empowerment efforts. However, night shift teams were not found to be successful unless their was a nucleus of permanent night shift direct care workers.

In NH facilities, there may be multiple teams per shift. For example, if there are multiple wings of the NH, with six or seven direct care workers assigned to each wing and with little crossover of direct care workers between wings, then it would be best to establish a team for each wing. In no case should a team be larger than about 10 direct care workers. Experience shows that when a team gets too large, some direct care workers will not participate at all in team activities (they typically attend the meeting, but their attention is elsewhere), and a small group of direct care workers will dominate the team's decision-making activities.

The managers and nurses should also identify a viable place for each of the teams to meet. This should be a place where the team has privacy. That is, no one, including managers, nurses, and residents, will be able to listen in on or disturb the direct care workers while they are meeting. Otherwise, during their meeting the direct care workers will be concerned about being overheard by management and nurses or being interrupted by residents. With regard to the day and time of the weekly team meetings, the direct care workers typically can be given this responsibility because they are in the best position to know the best time for them to meet. Occasionally, the team may experiment with one day and time and then determine that it is not working and try another.

8. *For each EWT, identify a manager or nurse who will be responsible for weekly communications with the team.* Each team will be taking weekly notes and submitting them to a manager or nurse. These notes will include what was covered during the weekly meeting, questions that team members have for management and nurses, answers to questions asked of the team by management and nurses, team suggestions for improving work procedures, and so on. It is important that one or more managers or nurses take responsibility for responding to the team each week and keeping the team involved in the workplace decisions being made by management. This might be the director of nursing, the assistant director of nursing, a nurse supervisor, or a combination of managers and nurses who meet each week and decide how to respond to the team and how to keep the team involved in decisions being made. Furthermore, for each additional EWT implemented, it is crucial to make clear which manager or nurse or combination thereof will be responsible for weekly communications with this newly implemented team. Without this kind of commitment and regular communication from management and nurses, the EWT members will become disillusioned, and the team will become ineffective.

9. *Determine the first decisions that EWTs will be allowed to participate in or make for themselves.* During the training process, managers and nurses can be encouraged to identify issues that the EWTs can take on. For example, an EWT may be asked to evaluate how meal trays are being distributed to residents and provide suggestions on how to revise the procedures so that all residents receive a meal while it is still hot. When implementing this step, it is important that management and nurses be prepared to provide the team with some background on the issue and any pertinent information. In particular, this should include the primary reason for focusing on the issue being brought to the team, whether due to complaints from family or residents, a deficiency identified from a health survey, or a desire to improve before one of the first two occurs. Management and nurses should also provide any important information that the team may need in order to make the best decision.

Similarly, during the training process the members of an EWT can be asked to identify work procedures or other issues that they believe are important and need attention. The trainer can take this to the managers and nurses to determine whether they want to give the team the go-ahead for examining the issue. If they agree, they might also provide the team with any relevant information that will help them to make the best decisions or develop the most effective work procedures.

10. *One or two EWTs begin holding weekly meetings.* EWTs typically hold at least one 30-minute sit-down meeting a week. The EWTs that received the in-depth training should have already been instructed to choose a day and time to meet that appeared best (e.g., a slow time during their work shift). All team members on duty

should attend the meeting, and while they are meeting nurses should cover their duties such as answering resident call lights.

During or before the first meeting, the direct care workers should choose a team leader and a backup team leader. Their responsibilities are described in Chapter 11. In some cases the team may choose to rotate the team leader position, and in others the team may choose to have co–team leaders. In either case, the team should be free to change team leaders whenever the team members want to do so or when the team leader wants to relinquish the responsibility.

The trained team facilitator should attend and facilitate the weekly meetings. The facilitator should begin skipping the weekly team meetings and allowing the team to meet on its own as the weeks progress and the team members become more proficient at communication, cooperative conflict, problem solving, and decision making (see Chapter 11). Eventually, the team facilitator will act more as a consultant to the team than a facilitator. That is, the team will contact the facilitator or invite the facilitator to their meeting when they feel the need for help. Otherwise, the facilitator will rarely attend the EWT's meetings.

It is beneficial if the first team meetings double as training sessions for the direct care workers. That is, the team training session could occur on the same day and time and in the same location where the team's weekly meetings are planned to occur. This will allow the direct care workers to become accustomed to meeting on this particular day and time and to getting their work caught up before the meetings and training sessions so that they leave as little work as possible for the nurses who will be covering for them while they are meeting. Furthermore, providing training in a team meeting environment can facilitate the training of interpersonal skills, which our experience showed was provided most effectively as on-the-job training. That is, as the direct care workers interact during their training, the facilitator may gently note when a lack of interpersonal skills is displayed (e.g., making fun of someone's suggestion, not listening to others, verbally attacking another direct care worker) and when interpersonal skills are being used effectively (e.g., asking for others' opinions, showing respect for others who have different opinions). Once the training sessions are complete, the team will continue to meet at the same day and time, but the team trainer will no longer be present, and the team facilitator will assist the team in following its agenda (see Chapter 11).

11. *The EWT begins participating in decision making.* Once they complete their training and continue to meet on a regular basis, the EWT can begin reviewing workplace issues and procedures and making recommendations to management. The specific issues and procedures may be given to them by management and nurses or may be identified by a team member (see the Appendix Exhibit). Once a potential solution is selected by a team, it can be presented to the appropriate management person. This is typically the manager who presented the issue to the team or, if the issue originated from the team, the manager who is most directly associated with the issue. The manager then reviews the team's potential solution and as soon as possible provides feedback to the team. The manager may choose to accept the team solution as is, may suggest some changes to it, or may point out

serious shortcomings of the solution. In the latter case, the team typically is lacking some crucial information. When the team lacks information, the manager must take responsibility for providing the team with the information and then allow the team to reassess its solution with this additional information in hand (see Chapter 10).

It is crucial that management always be supportive of the team during this "play ball" process. Even poor choices by the team are likely to have some merits that can be highlighted. Furthermore, it is important that management not have a solution already in mind and force the team to continue reconsidering solutions until the solution matches that of management. In this situation, the team members soon recognize that it does not matter how seriously they take the problem or how hard they work to find a solution; whatever they propose will be rejected until it reflects what the manager wants. This quickly results in a team that stops problem solving. It is also valuable for managers to allow teams to try their solutions even when the solutions do not appear to be workable, as long as the solution will not harm a resident or have other significant adverse effects. Teams can grow substantially by being allowed to make mistakes, recognize them, and make corrections.

12. *New EWTs are trained and implemented.* Once one or two EWTs have been implemented and are performing at a high level, one or two additional EWTs can be implemented. All the preceding steps should be taken during this implementation process. Perhaps of most importance is the need to identify a manager or group of managers who agree to take responsibility for communicating with the new team. This includes responding to their suggestions and reading and responding to the team's notes each week.

Appendix Exhibit. An Example Topic Identified by an Empowered Work Team and Presented to Nurse Management

Several EWTs have identified "call-ins" as an issue important to the team and to the organization as a whole. Call-ins are team members who call in, typically at the beginning of a shift, to report that they will be absent from work that day (or night) or will be late arriving to work. These EWTs reported to management that call-ins by team members mess up the team's schedule and produce problems throughout the work day. The teams recognized that when a team member is ill, a call-in is necessary. However, they noted the need to discourage unnecessary call-ins. The teams offered several options for dealing with call-ins. These included the following:

- If a direct care worker misses work three times in 2 weeks without a good reason (e.g., a note from a doctor) or if the direct care worker is routinely absent, he or she should be suspended from work for a set period of time without the opportunity to make up the lost hours of work.

- If a person routinely comes in to work late, on the fourth time she or he should be sent home and not allowed to work that day, without the opportunity to make up the lost hours of work.

- The team supervisor should set an example by not being routinely absent or tardy.

- If the direct care worker calls in and says that he or she will be late but then does not come in and does not call back to let everyone know that he or she will not be coming in, then the person should be suspended.

- Those who call in frequently should not be allowed to do double shifts to make up for lost work time.

- Management should keep personal reasons for absences or tardiness confidential.

- Perfect attendance should be rewarded, such as with some sort of bonus (e.g., cash, small gift, certificate to a store or restaurant).

References and Suggested Readings

The 2006 Overview of Assisted Living. (2006). Washington, DC: American Association of Housing and Services for the Aging, American Seniors Housing Association, Assisted Living Federation of America, National Center for Assisted Living, National Investment Center.

Alecxih, L.M.B., Lutzky, S., Corea, J., & Coleman, B. (1996). *Estimated savings from the use of home and community-based alternatives to nursing facility care in three states.* Washington, DC: AARP, Public Policy Institute.

American Health Care Association. (2003). *Results of the 2002 AHCA survey of nursing staff vacancy and turnover in nursing homes.* Retrieved July 1, 2007, from http://www.ahca.org/research/rpt_vts2002_final.pdf

Ancona, D.G., & Caldwell, D.F. (1992). Bridging the boundary: External activity and performance in organizational teams. *Administrative Science Quarterly, 37,* 634–665.

Anderson, C.A. (1992, November). Total quality in practice: There are few (if any) universal truths. *Quality Matters,* pp. 6–7.

Anderson, R.A., & McDaniel, R.R. (1998). Intensity of registered nurse participation in nursing home decision making. *The Gerontologist, 38*(1), 90–100.

Anthony, W.P. (1978). *Participative management.* Reading, MA: Addison-Wesley.

Baguey, K. (1999). Workplace empowerment, job strain, and affective organizational commitment in critical care nurses: Testing Kanter's structural theory of organizational behavior. *JONA, 31,* 271.

Banaszak-Holl, J., & Hines, M.A. (1996). Factors associated with nursing home staff turnover. *The Gerontologist, 36,* 512–517.

Bandura, A. (1997). *Self-efficacy.* New York: Freeman.

Barba, B., Tesh, A., & Courts, N. (2002). Promoting thriving in nursing homes: The Eden alternative. *Journal of Gerontological Nursing, 28*(3), 7–13.

Barber, C., & Iwai, M. (1996). Role conflict and role ambiguity as predictors of burnout among staff caring for elderly dementia patients. *Journal of Gerontological Social Work, 26*(1/2), 101–116.

Barrick, A.L., Rader, J., Hoeffer, B., & Sloane, P.D. (Eds.). (2000). Bathing without a battle: Personal care of individuals with dementia. *The Gerontologist, 46,* 532.

Beck, C., Ortigara, A., Mercer, S., & Shue, V. (1999). Enabling and empowering certified nursing assistants for quality dementia care. *International Journal of Geriatric Psychiatry, 14,* 197–212.

Becker-Reems, E.D. (1994). *Self-managed work teams in health care organizations.* Chicago: American Hospital Publications.

Belasco, J., & Stayer, R. (1994). Why empowerment doesn't empower. *Business Horizons, 37*(2), 29–42.

Beyerlein, M., & Johnson, D. (1994). *Advances in interdisciplinary studies of work teams.* Volume 1. *1994: Theories of self-managing teams.* Greenwich, CT: JAI Press.

Bielby, W.T., & Bielby, D.D. (1989). Family ties: Balancing commitments to work and family in dual earner households. *American Sociological Review, 54,* 776–789.

Binstock, R.H., & Spector, W.D. (1997, December). Five priority areas for research on long-term care. *Health Services Research, 32*(5), 715–730.

Bishop, C. (2004). Paid home care in the 21st century: Need and demand. *Home Health Care Management & Practice, 16,* 350–359.

Black, J.S., & Gregersen, H.B. (1997). Participative decision-making: An integration of multiple dimensions. *Human Relations, 50*(7), 859–878.

Bliesmer, M., & Earle, P. (1993, June). Research considerations. *Journal of Gerontological Nursing,* pp. 27–34.

Bouckaert, L. (1999). The ethics of participation. *Journal of Business Ethics, 21,* 95–96.

Bowen, D., & Lawler, E. (1992, Spring). The empowerment of service workers. *Sloan Management Review,* pp. 31–39.

Bowers, B., & Becker, M. (1992). Nurse's aides in nursing homes: The relationship between organization and quality. *The Gerontologist, 32,* 360–366.

Bowers, B.J., Faan, S.E., & Jacobson, N. (2003, March). Turnover reinterpreted. *Journal of Gerontological Nursing,* pp. 36–43.

Brannon, D., Zinn, J.S., Mor, V., & Davis, J. (2002). An exploration of job, organizational, and environmental factors associated with high and low nursing assistant turnover. *The Gerontologist, 42,* 159–168.

Brightman, H.J. (1988). *Group problem solving: An improved managerial approach.* Atlanta: Georgia State University Business Publishing Division.

Brod, M., Stewart, A.L., Sands, L., & Walton, P. (1999). Conceptualization and measurement of quality of life in dementia: The Dementia Quality of Life instrument (DQoL). *The Gerontologist, 39*(1), 25–35.

Brown, E.L., Raue, P.J., Mlodzianowski, A.E., Meyers, B.S., Greenberg, R.L., & Bruce, M.L. (2006). Transition to home care: Quality of mental health, pharmacy, and medical history information. *International Journal of Psychiatry in Medicine, 36*(3), 339–349.

Brunk, D. (1997). Random acts of violence. *Contemporary Long Term Care,* 38–42.

Buhler-Wilkerson, K. (2001). *No place like home: A history of nursing and home care in the United States.* Baltimore: Johns Hopkins University Press.

Burgio, L., Lichstein, K.L., Nichols, L., Czaja, S., Gallagher-Thompson, D., Bourgeois, M., et al. (2001). Judging outcomes in psychosocial interventions for dementia caregivers: The problem of treatment implementation. *The Gerontologist, 41,* 481–489.

Campbell, D.T., & Stanley, J. (1966). *Experimental and quasi-experimental designs for research.* Chicago: Rand McNally.

Campion, M.A., Medsker, G.J., & Higgs, A.C. (1993). Relations between work group characteristics and effectiveness: Implications for designing effective work groups. *Personnel Psychology, 46,* 823–850.

Carder, P.C., Morgan, L.A., & Eckert, J.K. (2005). Small board-and-care homes in the age of assisted living. *Generations, 29*(4), 24–31.

Castle, N.G. (2006). Measuring staff turnover in nursing homes. *The Gerontologist, 46,* 210–219.

Castle, N.G. (2007). Assessing job satisfaction of nurse aides in nursing homes. *Journal of Gerontological Nursing, 33*(5), 41–47.

Castle, N.G., & Engberg, J. (2006). Organizational characteristics associated with staff turnover in nursing homes. *The Gerontologist, 46,* 62–73.

Castle, N.G., Engberg, J., Anderson, R., & Men, A. (2007). Job satisfaction of nurse aides in nursing homes: Intent to leave and turnover. *The Gerontologist, 47,* 193–204.

Caudill, M.E., & Patrick, M. (1991–1992). Turnover among nursing assistants: Why they leave and why they stay. *The Journal of Long-Term Care Administration, 19*(4), 29–32.

Centers for Disease Control. (2004). *Current home health care patients.* Retrieved January 19, 2007, from http://www.cdc.gov/nchs/data/nhhcsd/currhomecare00

Centers for Medicare and Medicaid Services. (2000). *Report to Congress: Appropriateness of minimum nurse staffing ratios in nursing homes. Phase I report. U.S. Department of Health and Human Services.* Retrieved July 1, 2007, from http://www.cms.gov/medicaid

Coburn, A.F., Fralich, J.T., McGuire, C., & Fortinsky, R.H. (1996, June). Variations in outcomes of care in urban and rural nursing facilities in Maine. *Journal of Applied Gerontology, 15*(2), 202–223.

Cohen, S.G. (1994). Designing effective self-managing work teams. In M.M. Beyerlein & D.A. Johnson (Eds.), *Advances in interdisciplinary studies of work teams: Theories of self-managed work teams* (pp. 67–102). London: JAI Press.

Cohen-Mansfield, J. (1997). Turnover among nursing home staff: A review. *Nursing Management, 28*(5), 59–64.

Cohen-Mansfield, J., Ejaz, F.K., & Werner, P. (2000). *Satisfaction surveys in long-term care.* New York: Springer.

Cohen-Mansfield, J., & Noelker, L. (2000). Nursing staff satisfaction in long-term care. In J. Cohen-Mansfield, F.K. Ejaz, & P. Werner (Eds.), *Satisfaction surveys in long-term care* (pp. 52–75). New York: Springer.

Cook, J.D., Hepworth, S.J., Wall, T.D., & Warr, P.B. (1979). *The experience of work.* New York: Academic Press.

Cotton, J.L., Vollrath, D.A., Froggatt, K.L., Lengnick-Hall, M.L., & Jennings, K.R. (1988). Employee participation: Diverse forms and different outcomes. *Academy of Management Review, 13*(1), 8–22.

Craft Morgan, J., & Conrad, T.R. (2007, January). *A mixed method evaluation of a workforce development intervention for nursing assistants in nursing homes: The case of WIN A STEP UP.* Discussion group, University of North Carolina, Chapel Hill.

Cummings, T.G. (1978). Self-regulating work groups: A socio-technical synthesis. *Academy of Management Review, 3*(3), 625–634.

Dale, S.B., & Brown, R. (2006). Reducing nursing home use through consumer-directed personal care services. *Medical Care, 44,* 760–767.

Dale, S., Brown, R., Phillips, B., Schore, J., & Carlson, B.L. (2003). The effects of cash and counseling on personal care services and Medicaid costs in Arkansas. *Health Affairs, W3,* 566–575.

Davis, M.A. (1991). On nursing home quality: A review and analysis. *Medical Care Review, 48*(1), 129–166.

Davis, M.A., Sebastian, J.G., & Tschetter, J. (1997). Measuring quality of nursing home service. *Psychological Reports, 81,* 531–542.

DeFrancis, M. (2002, January). U.S. elder care is in a fragile state. *Population Today, 30*(1), 4–7.

Deming, W.E. (1982). *Out of the crises.* Cambridge, MA: MIT Center for Advanced Engineering Study.

Department of Defense. (1994). *Self-managed work teams: Master plan.* St. Louis, MO: Defense Contract Management Office.

Department of Health and Human Services Office of the Assistant Secretary for Planning and Evaluation, Centers for Medicare and Medicaid Services, and Health Resource and Services Administration; and Department of Labor Office of the Assistant Secretary for Policy, Bureau of Labor Statistics, and Employment and Training Administration.

(2003). *The future supply of long-term care workers in relation to the aging baby boom generation: Report to Congress.* Washington, DC: Author.

Donoghue, C., & Castle, N.G. (2006). Voluntary and involuntary nursing home staff turnover. *Research on Aging, 28,* 454–472.

Donovan, M. (1988). Employees who manage themselves. *Journal for Quality and Participation, 11*(1), 58–61.

Donovan, M. (1989, December). Redesigning the workplace. *The Journal for Quality and Participation, 12*(Special Supplement), 6–8.

Doty, P. (2000). *Cost-effectiveness of home and community-based long-term care services.* USHHS/ASPE Office of Disability, Aging and Long-Term Care Policy. Retrieved June 6, 2001, from http://aspe.hhs.gov/daltcp/reports/costeff.htm

Eaton, S.C. (2000). Beyond "unloving care": Linking human resources management and patient care quality in nursing homes. *International Journal of Human Resources Management, 11,* 591–616.

Eaton, S.C. (2001, Winter). What a difference management makes! In Abt Associates (Ed.), *Appropriateness of minimum nurse staffing ratios in nursing homes.* Cambridge, MA: Abt Associates.

Ejaz, F.K. & Noelker, L.S. (2006). *Tailored and ongoing training can improve job satisfaction.* Cleveland, OH: Margaret Blenkner Research Institute, Benjamin Rose Institute.

Ejaz, F.K., Noelker, L.S., Menne, H.L., & Bagakas, J.G. (2008). The impact of stress and support on direct care workers' job satisfaction. *The Gerontologist, 48(1),* 60–70.

Fagan, R.M. (2003). Pioneer network. In A.S. Weiner & J.L. Ronch (Eds.), *Culture change in long-term care* (pp. 125–149). New York: Haworth.

Fisher, K., Rayner, S., & Belgard, W. (1995). *Tips for teams.* New York: McGraw-Hill.

Foner, N. (1994). Nursing home aides: Saints or monsters? *The Gerontologist, 34,* 245–250.

Ford, R.C., & Fottler, M.D. (1995). Empowerment: A matter of degree. *Academy of Management Executive, 9*(3), 21–31.

Foster, L., Brown, R., Phillips, B., & Carlson, B.L. (2005). Easing the burden of caregiving: The impact of consumer direction on primary informal caregivers in Arkansas. *The Gerontologist, 45,* 474–485.

Friedman, S., Daub, C., Cresci, K., & Keyser, R. (1999). A comparison of job satisfaction among nursing assistants in nursing homes and the Program of All-Inclusive Care for the Elderly (PACE). *The Gerontologist, 39*(4), 434–439.

Frost, C.H., Wakely, J., & Ruh, R.A. (1974). *The Scanlon plan for organization development: Identity, participation, and equity.* East Lansing: Michigan State University Press.

Galbraith, J. (1973). *Designing complex organizations.* Reading, MA: Addison-Wesley.

GAO. (1989). *Board and care: Insufficient assurances that residents' needs are identified and met* (GAO/HRD-89-50). Washington, DC: United State General Accounting Office.

GAO. (1992). *Board and care homes: Elderly at risk from mishandled medications* (GAO/HRD-92-45). Washington, DC: United States General Accounting Office.

Garrard, J.L., Buchanan, J.L., Ratner, E.R., Makris, L., Chan, H.C., Skay, C., et al. (1993). Differences between nursing home admissions and residents. *The Gerontologist, 40,* 671.

Gaugler, J.E., Kane, R.A., & Langlois, J. (2000). Assessment of family caregivers of older adults. In R.L. Kane & R.A. Kane (Eds.), *Assessing the well-being of older people: Measures, meaning, and practical applications* (pp. 320–359). New York: Oxford University Press.

Gaugler, J.E., & Teaster, P. (2006). The family caregiving career: Implications for community-based long-term care practice and policy. *Journal of Aging & Social Policy, 18,* 141–154.

Gilster, S.D., Accorinti, K.L., & Dalessandro, J.L. (2002). Providing a continuum of care for persons with Alzheimer's disease. *Alzheimer's Care Quarterly, 3*(2), 103–115.

Gladstein, D.L. (1984). Groups in context: A model of task group effectiveness. *Administrative Science Quarterly, 29*(4), 499–517.

Grant, L.A., Kane, R.A., Potthoff, S.J., & Ryden, M. (1996). Staff training and turnover in Alzheimer special care units: Comparisons with non–special care units. *Geriatric Nursing, 17,* 278–282.

Grant, L.A., & Norton, L. (2003, November). A stage model of culture change in nursing facilities. In *Culture change II: Theory and practice, vision and reality.* San Diego, CA: Gerontological Society of America.

Grau, L., Chandler, B., Burton, B., & Kolditz, D. (1991). Institutional loyalty and job satisfaction among nurse aides in nursing homes. *Journal of Aging and Health, 3,* 47–65.

Green House Project. (n.d.). Retrieved April 1, 2006, from http://www.edenalt.com

Griffin, R.W. (1988). Consequences of quality circles in an industrial setting: A longitudinal assessment. *Academy of Management Journal, 31*(2), 338–358.

Gross, S.E. (1995). *Compensation for teams: How to design and implement team-based reward programs.* New York: AMACOM.

Hackman, J.R. (1978). The design of self-managing work groups. In S. Biking, S. Streufert, & F.E. Fiedler (Eds.), *Managerial control and organizational democracy* (pp. 61–91). New York: Wiley.

Hackman, J.R. (1988). The design of work teams. In J.W. Lorsch (Ed.), *Handbook of organizational behavior* (pp. 315–342). Englewood Cliffs, NJ: Prentice Hall.

Hackman, J.R. (1990). *Groups that work (and those that don't).* San Francisco: Jossey-Bass.

Hackman, J.R., & Oldham, G.R. (1976). Motivation through the design of work: Test of a theory. *Organizational Behavior and Human Performance, 16,* 250–279.

Hackman, J.R., & Oldham, G.R. (1980). *Work redesign.* Reading, MA: Addison-Wesley.

Halbur, B. (1986). Managing nursing personnel turnover rates: Strategies for nursing home professionals. *Journal of Applied Gerontology, 5*(1), 64–75.

Han, B., Sirrocco, A., & Rembsburg, R. (2003). *Developing a typology of long-term care residential places: The first step.* Washington, DC: Long-Term Care Statistical Branch, Division of Health Care Statistics, National Center for Health Statistics.

Harrington, C., Chapman, S., Miller, E., Miller, N., & Newcomer, R.J. (2005). Trends in the supply of long-term-care facilities and beds in the U.S. *Journal of Applied Gerontology, 24*(4), 265–282.

Harrington, C., Kovner, C., Mezey, M., Kayser-Jones, J., Burger, S., Mohler, M., et al. (2000). Experts recommend minimum nurse staffing standards for nursing facilities in the United States. *The Gerontologist, 40,* 5–16.

Harrington, C., & Swan, J.H. (2003). Nursing home staffing, turnover, and case mix. *Medical Care Research and Review, 60,* 366–392.

Harrington, C., Zimmerman, D., Karon, S.L., Robinson, J., & Beutel, P. (2000). Nursing home staffing and its relationship to deficiencies. *The Journals of Gerontology, 55B,* S278–S287.

Hawes, C., Phillips, C.D., & Rose, M.S. (2000). *High service or high privacy assisted living facilities, their residents and staff: Results from a national survey.* U.S. Department of Health and Human Services. Retrieved December 8, 2002, from http://aspe.hhs.gov/daltcp/reports/hshp.htm

Hawes, C., Phillips, C.D., Rose, M., Holan, S., & Sherman, M. (2003). A national survey of assisted living facilities. *The Gerontologist, 43*(6), 875–882.

Hawes, C., Rose, M., & Phillips, C.D. (1999). *A national study of assisted living for the frail elderly: Results of a national survey of facilities.* Washington, DC: U.S. Department of Health and Human Services.

Health Care Financing Administration. (2000). *Medicare 2000*. Washington, DC: Government Printing Office.

Hedrick, S.C., Sales, A.E., Sullivan, J.H., Gray, S.L., Tornatore, J., Curtis, M., et al. (2003). Resident outcomes of Medicaid-funded community residential care. *The Gerontologist, 43*(4), 473–482.

Heiselman, T., & Noelker, L.S. (1991). Enhancing mutual respect among nursing assistants, residents, and residents' families. *The Gerontologist, 31*(4), 552–555.

Helmer, F.T., Olson, S.F., & Heim, R.I. (1993). Strategies for nurse job satisfaction. *The Journal of Long-Term Care Administration, 21*(2), 10–14.

Henricks, M. (1997, May). Golden rules. *Entrepreneur*, pp. 147–151.

Hepburn, K.W., & Keenan, J.M. (1997). The role of the physician in home care. In M.D. Harris (Ed.), *Handbook of home health care administration* (2nd ed., pp. 823–830). Gaithersburg, MD: Aspen.

Hernandez, M. (2006). Assisted living in all of its guises. *Generations, 29*(4), 16–23.

Hitchcock, D., & Willard, M. (1995). *Why teams can fail and what to do about it: Essential tools for anyone implementing self-directed work teams*. Chicago: Irwin.

Hoeffer, B., Talerico, K.A., Rasin, J., Mitchell, M., Stewart, B.J., McKenzie, D., et al. (2006). Assisting cognitively impaired nursing home residents with bathing: Effects of two bathing interventions on caregiving. *The Gerontologist, 46*, 524–532.

Hollinger-Smith, L. (2003). It takes a village to retain quality nursing staff: The Mather LifeWays LEAP training program uses the three Rs of retention to prevent staff turnover. *Nursing Homes Magazine, 52*(5), 52–54.

Hollinger-Smith, L.M., Lindeman, D., Leary, M., & Ortigara, A. (2002). Building the foundation for quality improvement: LEAP for a quality long-term care workforce. *Senior Housing and Care Journal 10*, 31–43.

Hollinger-Smith, L., Ortigara, A., & Lindeman, D. (2001). Developing a comprehensive long term care workforce initiative. *Alzheimer's Care Quarterly, 2*(3), 33–40.

Holt, D.H. (1990). *Management: Principles and practices*. Englewood Cliffs, NJ: Prentice Hall.

Hyman, J., & Mason, B. (1995). *Managing employee involvement and participation*. Thousand Oaks, CA: Sage.

Ilgen, D.R., & Klein, H.J. (1988). Individual motivation and performance: Cognitive influences on effort and choice. In J.P. Campbell, R.J. Campbell, & Associates (Eds.), *Productivity in organizations: New perspectives from industrial and organizational psychology* (pp. 143–176). San Francisco: Jossey-Bass.

Institute of Medicine. (1986). *Improving the quality of care in nursing homes*. Washington, DC: National Academy Press.

Institute of Medicine. (2001). *Improving the quality of long-term care*. Washington, DC: National Academy Press.

Irvine, D.M., & Evans, M.G. (1995). Job satisfaction and turnover among nurses: Integrating research findings across studies. *Nursing Research, 44*, 246–253.

Jewell, L., & Reitz, J. (1988). Group decision making. In R. Katz (Ed.), *Managing professionals in innovative organizations* (pp. 247–261). Cambridge, MA: Ballinger.

Johnson, D.W., & Johnson, F.P. (1994). *Joining together: Group theory and group skills* (3rd ed.). Upper Saddle River, NJ: Prentice Hall.

Kane, R.A. (2001). Long-term care and a good quality of life: Bringing them closer together. *The Gerontologist, 41*(3), 293–304.

Kane, R.A., Caplan, A.L., Urv-Wong, E.K., Freeman, I.C., Aroskar, M.A., & Finch, M. (1997). Everyday matters in the lives of nursing home residents: Wish for and perception of choice and control. *Journal of the American Geriatrics Society, 45*, 1086–1093.

Kane, R.A., Lum, T.Y., Cutler, L.J., Degenholtz, H.B., & Yu, T.-C. (2007). Resident outcomes in small-house nursing homes: A longitudinal evaluation of the initial Green House Program. *Journal of the American Geriatric Society, 55*, 832–839.

Kane, R.A., & Wilson, K.B. (1993). *Assisted living in the United States: A new paradigm for residential care.* Washington, DC: American Association of Retired Persons.

Kane, R.A., & Wilson, K.B. (2001). *Assisted living at the crossroads: principles for its future* (discussion paper). Portland, OR: Jessie F. Richardson Foundation.

Kanter, R.M. (1993). Men and women of the corporation. *JONA, 31*, 271.

Kash, B.A., Castle, N.G., Naufal, G.S., & Hawes, C. (2006). Effect of staff turnover on staffing: A closer look at registered nurses, licensed vocational nurses, and certified nursing assistants. *The Gerontologist, 46*, 609–619.

Katz, D., & Kahn, R. (1966). *The social psychology of organizations.* New York: Wiley.

Kayser-Jones, J., & Schell, E.S. (1997). Staffing and the mealtime experience of nursing residents on a special care unit. *American Journal of Alzheimer's Disease and Other Dementias, 12*, 67–72.

Kayser-Jones, J., Schell, E.S., Porter, C., Barbaccia, J.C., & Shaw, H. (1999). Factors contributing to dehydration in nursing homes: Inadequate staffing and lack of professional supervision. *Journal of the American Geriatrics Society, 47*, 1187–1194.

Keane, B. (2004, August). Building the new culture of aging one leader at a time. *Nursing Homes, 53*(8), 44.

Kehoe, M.A., & Heesch, B.V. (2003). Culture change in long term care. In A.S. Weiner & J. Ronch (Eds.), *Culture change in long-term care* (pp. 159–174). New York: Haworth.

Kelly, M. (1991). *The adventures of a self-managing team.* San Diego, CA: Pfeiffer.

Kettlitz, G. (1998). Validity of background data as a predictor of employee tenure among nursing aides in long-term care facilities. *Health Care Supervisor, 16*(3), 26–31.

Kirkman, B.L., & Rosen, B. (1999). Beyond self-management: Antecedents and consequences of team empowerment. *Academy of Management Journal, 42*(1), 58–74.

Kleinsorge, I.K., & Koenig, H.F. (1991). The silent customers. *Journal of Health Care Marketing, 11*(4), 2–14.

Kovach, C.R., & Krejci, J.W. (1998). Facilitating change in dementia care. *Journal of Nursing Administration, 28*(5), 17–27.

Kovach, C.R., & Meyer-Arnold, E.A. (1996). Coping with conflicting agendas: The bathing experience of cognitively impaired older adults. *The Gerontologist, 46*, 532.

Kren, L. (1992). Budgetary participation and managerial performance: The impact of information and environmental volatility. *The Accounting Review, 67*(3), 511–526.

Kruzich, J.M., Clinton, J.F., & Kelber, S.T. (1992). Personal and environmental influences on nursing home satisfaction. *The Gerontologist, 32*(3), 342–350.

Lambert, S. (1990). Processes linking work and family: A critical review and research agenda. *Human Relations, 43*(3), 239–257.

Landy, F.J., & Becker, W.S. (1987). Motivation theory reconsidered. *Research in Organizational Behavior, 9*, 1–38.

Laschinger, H.K.S., Finegan, J., Shamian, J., & Casier, S. (2000). Organizational trust and empowerment in restructured health care settings: Effects on staff nurse commitment. *JONA, 31*, 271.

Laschinger, H.K.S., Finegan, J., Shamian, J., & Wills, P. (2001). Impact of structural and psychological empowerment on job strain in nursing work settings: Expanding Kanter's model. *JONA, 31*, 260.

Laschinger, H.K.S., & Havens, D.S. (1996). Staff nurse empowerment and perceived control over nursing practice. *JONA, 31*, 271.

Laschinger, H.K.S., Wong, C., McMahon, L., & Kaufmann, C. (1999). Leader behaviour impact on staff nurse empowerment, job tension and work effectiveness. *JONA*, *31*, 271.

Lawler, E.E. III. (1986). *High-involvement management*. San Francisco: Jossey-Bass.

Lawler, E.E. III. (1989). Substitutes for hierarchy. *Incentive*, *163*(3), 39–45.

Lawler, E.E. III. (1992). *The ultimate advantage: Creating the high involvement organization*. San Francisco: Jossey-Bass.

Lawler, E.E. III, & Mohrman, S.A. (1987). Quality circles: After the honeymoon. *Organizational Dynamics*, *15*(4), 42–54.

Lekan-Rutledge, D., Palmer, M.H., & Belyea, M. (1998). In their own words: Nursing assistants' perceptions of barriers to implementation of prompted voiding in long-term care. *The Gerontologist*, *38*(3), 370–378.

Likert, R.L. (1967). *The human organization*. New York: McGraw-Hill.

Locke, E.A., & Latham, G. (1990). Work motivation and satisfaction: Light at the end of the tunnel. *American Psychological Society*, *1*(4), 240–246.

Locke, E.A., & Schweiger, D.M. (1979). Participation in decision-making: One more look. In B.M. Staw (Ed.), *Research in organizational behavior* (pp. 265–339). Greenwich: JAI Press.

Logsdon, R.G., Gibbons, L.E., McCurry, S.M., & Teri, L. (1999). Quality of life in Alzheimer's disease: Patient and caregiver reports. *Journal of Mental Health and Aging*, *5*, 21–32.

Lustbader, W. (2001). The Pioneer challenge: A radical change in the culture of nursing homes. In L.S. Noelker & Z. Harel (Eds.), *Linking quality of long-term care and quality of life* (pp. 185–203). New York: Springer.

Macy, B.A., Peterson, M.F., & Norton, L.W. (1989). A test of participation theory in a work re-design field setting: Degree of participation and comparison site contrasts. *Human Relations*, *42*(12), 1095–1165.

Magaziner, J., German, P., Zimmerman, S.I., Hebel, J.R., Burton, L., Gruber-Baldini, A.L., et al. (2000). The prevalence of dementia in a statewide sample of new nursing home admissions age 65 and over: Diagnosis by expert panel. *The Gerontologist*, *40*, 663–672.

Maier, G. (2002). Career ladders: An important element in CNA retention. *Geriatric Nursing*, *23*, 217–219.

Manz, C.C., & Sims, H.P., Jr. (1987). Leading workers to lead themselves: The external leadership of self-managing work teams. *Administrative Science Quarterly*, *32*, 106–128.

Maslach, C., Jackson, S.E., & Leiter, M.P. (1996). *Maslach burnout inventory manual* (3rd ed.). Palo Alto, CA: Consulting Psychologists Press.

May, B.J. (1999). *Home health and rehabilitation: Concepts of care* (2nd ed.). Philadelphia: F.A. Davis.

McDonald, C. (1991–1992). Career ladder: Tool for recruitment, retention, and recognition. *Journal Lab*, pp. 6–7.

McGee, G., & Ford, R.C. (1987). Two (or more) dimensions of organizational commitment: Reexamination of the affective and continuance commitment scales. *Journal of Applied Psychology*, *72*(4), 638–642.

McGrath, J.E. (1964). *Social psychology: A brief introduction*. Englewood Cliffs, NJ: Prentice Hall.

Menne, H.L., Noelker, L.S., Ejaz, F.K., & Fox, K.M. (2006, November). *The importance of organizational practices and personal characteristics on nursing assistant job satisfaction*. Poster presented at the Gerontological Society of America conference, Dallas, TX.

MetLife. (2005). *The MetLife market survey of assisted living costs*. Westport, CT: MetLife Mature Market Institute.

Miller, K.I., & Monge, P.R. (1986). Participation, satisfaction, and productivity: A meta-analytic review. *Academy of Management Journal, 29*(4), 727–753.

Mobley, W.H., Griffeth, R.W., Hand, H.H., & Meglino, B.M. (1979). Review and conceptual analysis of the employee turnover process. *Psychological Bulletin, 86*(3), 493–522.

Mollica, R., & Johnson-Lamarche, H. (2005). *Residential care and assisted living compendium 2004*. Washington, DC: Department of Health and Human Services, Office of Assistant Secretary for Planning and Evaluation.

Montgomery, R.J.V., Holley, L., Deichert, J., & Kosloski, K. (2005). A profile of home care workers from the 2000 census: How it changes what we know. *The Gerontologist, 45*(5), 593–600.

Morris, R., Caro, F., & Hansan, J. (1998). *Personal assistance: The future of home care*. Baltimore: Johns Hopkins University Press.

Myers, M.S. (1991). *Every employee a manager*. San Diego: University Assoc.

Nakhnikian, E., Wilner, M.A., & Hurd, D. (2002). Nursing assistant training and education: Recommendations for change. *Nursing Homes Magazine*, pp. 44–47.

National Association for Home Care and Hospice. (2007). *What types of services do home care providers deliver?* Retrieved January 19, 2007, from http://www.nahc.org/famcar_types

National Center for Assisted Living. (2007). *Assisted living state regulatory review*. Washington, DC: Author.

Navarra, T., & Ferrer, M.L. (1997). *An insider's guide to home health care*. Thorofare, NJ: Slack.

Neuhaus, R.H. (1990). *Long term care administration: Teamwork and effective management*. New York: University Press of America.

Newcomer, R.J., Breuer, W., & Zhang, X. (1994). *Residents and the appropriateness of placement in residential care for the elderly: a 1993 survey of California RCFE operators and residents*. San Francisco: Institute for Health & Aging, University of California San Francisco.

Newcomer, R., Flores, C., & Hernandez, M. (in press). Intended and unintended consequences of state and federal policies and regulations. In S. Gollant & J. Hyde (Eds.), *The assisted living residence: A vision for the future*. Baltimore: Johns Hopkins University Press.

Nieva, N.F., Fleishman, E.A., & Rieck, A. (1978). *Team dimensions: Their identity, their measurement, and their relationships*. Washington, DC: Advanced Research Resources Organizations.

Niewnhous, S. (2007). How does "quality" fit in "pay for performance"? *Home Health Care Management & Practice, 19*, 91–93.

Noble, M. (2004, January/February). A mentoring program to reduce turnover. *Best Practices*, pp. 11–13.

Noelker, L.S., & Ejaz, F.K. (2001). *Improving work settings and job outcomes for nursing assistants in skilled care facilities*. Final report submitted to the Cleveland Foundation and the Retirement Research Foundation.

Noelker, L.S., Ejaz, F.K., Menne, H.L., & Jones, J.A. (2006). The impact of stress and support on nursing assistant satisfaction with supervision. *Journal of Applied Gerontology, 25*, 307–323.

Nordheimer, J. (1995, April 10). A mature housing market: A growing business in not-quite-nursing-home care. *The New York Times*, pp. D1, 19.

Nurick, A. (1982). Participation in organizational change: A longitudinal field study. *Human Relations, 35*, 413–430.

Orsburn, J., Moran, L., Musselwhite, E., Zenger, J.H., & Perrin, C. (1990). *Self-directed work teams: The new American challenge*. Homewood, IL: Business One Irwin.

Packer-Tursman, J. (1996, February). Reversing the revolving door syndrome: How to find and keep quality care staff. *Provider*, pp. 51–54.

Pallarito, K. (1995, May 8). Assisted living captures profitable market niche. *Modern Healthcare*, pp. 73–75.

Paraprofessional Health Care Institute. (2003, May). Introducing peer mentoring in long-term care settings. *Workforce Strategies*, p. 2.

Parsons, S.K., Simmons, W.P., Penn, K., & Furlough, M. (2003). Determinants of satisfaction and turnover among nursing assistants. *Journal of Gerontological Nursing, 29*(3), 51–58.

Pasmore, W.A., Francis, C., Haldeman, J., & Shani, A. (1982). Sociotechnical systems: A North American reflection on empirical studies of the seventies. *Human Relations, 35*(12), 1179–1204.

Pasmore, W.A., & Purser, R.E. (1993, July–August). Designing work systems for knowledge workers. *Journal for Quality and Participation*.

Pearce, J.A. II, & Ravlin, E.C. (1987). The design and activation of self-regulating work groups. *Human Relations, 40*(11), 751–782.

Peters, D.A., & McKeon, T. (1998). *Transforming home care*. Gaithersburg, MD: Aspen.

Pillemer, K., Suitor, J.J., & Wethington, E. (2003). Integrating theory, basic research, and intervention. *The Gerontologist, 43*(Special Issue), 19–28.

Plunkett, L.C., & Fournier, R. (1991). *Participative management: Implementing empowerment*. New York: Wiley.

Potterfield, T.A. (1999). *The business of employee empowerment: Democracy and ideology in the workplace*. Westport, CT: Quorum.

Pratt, J.R. (2004). *Assisted living, long-term care: Managing across the continuum* (2nd ed., pp. 96–119). Sudbury, MA: Jones and Bartlett.

Price, J.L., & Mueller, C.W. (1981). A causal model of turnover for nurses. *Academy of Management Journal, 24*, 543–565.

Quadagno, J. (2002). *Aging and the life course*. New York: McGraw-Hill.

Quinn, J.B. (1992). *Intelligent enterprise*. New York: Free Press.

Quinn, R.P., & Staines, G.L. (1979). *The 1977 quality of employment survey*. Ann Arbor: University of Michigan Institute of Social Research.

Rabig, J., Thomas, W., Kane, R., Cutler, L., & McAlilly, S. (2006). Radical redesign of nursing homes: Applying the Green House concept in Tupelo, Mississippi. *The Gerontologist, 46*(4), 533–536.

Ray, D.W., & Bronstein, H. (1995). *Teaming up: Making the transition to a self-directed, team-based organization*. New York: McGraw-Hill.

Reinhard, S., & Stone, R. (2001). *Promoting quality in nursing homes*. Washington, DC: American Association of Homes and Services for the Aging.

Reinhard, S.C., Young, H.M., Kane, R.A., & Quinn, W.V. (2006). Nurse delegation of medication administration for older adults in assisted living. *Nursing Outlook, 54*(2), 74–80.

Remsburg, R.E., Armacost, K.A., & Bennett, R.G. (1999). Improving nursing assistant turnover and stability rates in a long-term care facility. *Geriatric Nursing, 20*, 203–208.

Rennecker, J.A. (1996). Team building for continuous quality improvement. *Seminars in Perioperative Nursing, 5*(1), 40–46.

Robertson, J.F., & Cummings, C.C. (1991). What makes long-term-care nursing attractive? *The American Journal of Nursing, 91*(11), 41–46.

Robinson, S.B., & Rosher, R.B. (2006). Tangling with the barriers to culture change: Creating a resident-centered nursing home environment. *Journal of Gerontological Nursing, 32*(10), 19–25.

Rosen, J., Mittal, V., Degenholtz, H., Castle, N., Mulsant, B., Rhee, Y., et al. (2005). Organizational change and quality improvement in nursing homes. *Journal of Health Care Quality, 27*(607–612), 6–14, 21, 44.

Rosenberg, M., Schooler, C., & Schoenbach, C. (1989, December). Self-esteem and adolescent problems. *American Sociological Review, 54,* 1004–1018.

Sagie, A., & Koslowsky, M. (2000). *Participation and empowerment in organizations: Modeling, effectiveness, and applications.* Thousand Oaks, CA: Sage.

Salas, E., Dickinson, T.L., Converse, S.A., & Tannenbaum, S.I. (1992). Toward an understanding of team performance and training. In R.W. Swezey & E. Salas (Eds.), *Teams: Their training and performance* (pp. 3–30). Stamford, CT: Ablex.

Salmon, J., Hyer, K., Hedgecock, D., Zayac, H., & Engh, B. (2004). *Florida assisted living research study: Facilities, residents, staff, training and liability insurance: Executive summary* (USF #30347). Tampa: Florida Policy Exchange Center, Center for Housing and Long-Term Care, University of South Florida.

Saxon, J. (2000). *Teamwork in the nursing home.* Unpublished doctoral dissertation, University of North Texas, College of Public Affairs and Community Service, Denton, TX.

Schindler, P.L., & Thomas, C.C. (1993). The structure of interpersonal trust in the workplace. *Psychological Reports, 73,* 563–573.

Schroder, H.M. (1963). Conceptual organization and group structure. In O.J. Harvey (Ed.), *Motivation and social interaction* (pp. 134–166). New York: Ronald Press.

Schuster, F.E., Morden, D.L., Baker, T.E., McKay, I.S., Dunning, K.E., & Hagan, C.M. (1997). Management practice, organization climate, and performance. *Journal of Applied Behavioral Science, 33*(2), 209–226.

Seashore, S.E. (1954). *Group cohesiveness in the industrial work group.* Ann Arbor: University of Michigan Press.

Seavey, D. (2004). *Cost of frontline turnover in long-term care.* Washington, DC: Institute for the Future of Aging Services. Retrieved July 1, 2007, from http://www.bjbc.org/content/docs/TOCostReport.pdf

Shields, S. (2004). *Meadowlark Hills.* Manhattan, KS: Manhattan Retirement Foundation.

Shonk, J.H. (1992). *Team-based organizations: Developing a successful team environment.* Homewood, IL: Business One, Irwin.

Sikorska, E. (1999). Organizational determinants of resident satisfaction with assisted living. *The Gerontologist, 39*(4), 450–456.

Sikorska-Simmons, E. (2005). Predictors of organizational commitment among staff in assisted living. *The Gerontologist, 45*(2), 196–205.

Sikorska-Simmons, E. (2006). Organizational culture and work-related attitudes among staff in assisted living. *Journal of Gerontological Nursing, 32*(2), 19–27.

Simon-Rusinowitz, L., Mahoney, K.J., Loughlin, D.M., & DeBarthe Sadler, M. (2005). Paying family caregivers: An effective policy option in the Arkansas Cash and Counseling Demonstration. *Marriage & Family Review, 37,* 83–105.

Sims, H.P., & Lorenzi, P. (1992). *The new leadership paradigm.* Newbury Park, CA: Sage.

Sims, H.P. Jr., & Manz, C.C. (1994). The leadership of self-managing work teams. In M.M. Beyerlein & D.A. Johnson (Eds.), *Advances in interdisciplinary studies of work teams: Theories of self-managed work teams* (pp. 187–200). London: JAI Press.

Singer, J.N. (1974). Participative decision-making about work: An overdue look at variables which mediate its effects. *Sociology of Work and Occupations, 1,* 347–371.

Smith, A.J. (1960). A developmental study of group processes. *Journal of Genetic Psychology, 97,* 29–39.

Smith, C. (2006). Engaging the emotional, financial, and physical ramifications of long-distance caregiving. *Home Health Care Management & Practice, 18,* 463–466.

Somers, M.J. (1995). Organizational commitment, turnover and absenteeism: An examination of direct and interaction effects. *Journal of Organizational Behavior, 16,* 49–58.

Spector, P.E. (1986). Perceived control by employees: A meta-analysis of studies concerning autonomy and participation at work. *Human Relations, 39*(11), 1005–1016.

Spector, P.E. (1997). *Job satisfaction.* Thousand Oaks, CA: Sage.

Spiegel, A. (1987). *Home health care* (2nd ed.). Owings Mills, MD: National Health Publishing.

Spreitzer, G. (1995). Psychological empowerment in the workplace. *Academy of Management Journal, 38*(5), 1442–1465.

Spreitzer, G., Kizilos, M.A., & Nason, S.W. (1997). A dimensional analysis of the relationship between psychological empowerment and effectiveness, satisfaction, and strain. *Journal of Management, 23*(5), 679–704.

StataCorp. (2003). *Stata base reference manual* (Vol. 2, G-M, Release 8). College Station, TX: Stata Corporation.

Stearns, S.C., & Morgan, L.A. (2001). Economics and financing. In S. Zimmerman, P.D. Sloane, & J.K. Eckert (Eds.), *Assisted living: Needs, practices, and policies in residential care for the elderly* (pp. 271–291). Baltimore, MD: Johns Hopkins University Press.

Steers, R.M., & Spencer, D.G. (1977). The role of achievement motivation in job design. *Journal of Applied Psychology, 62,* 472–479.

Stein, R. (2001). Home-based comprehensive care services for children with chronic conditions. *Children's Services: Social Policy, Research, and Practice, 4*(4), 189–201.

Steiner, I.D. (1972). *Group processes and productivity.* New York: Academic Press.

Stewart, G.L., Carson, K.P., & Cardy, R.L. (1996, Spring). The joint effects of conscientiousness and self-leadership training on employee self-directed behavior in a service setting. *Personnel Psychology, 49*(1), 143–164.

Stone, R.I. (2004). The direct care worker: The third rail of home care policy. *Annual Review of Public Health, 25,* 521–537.

Stone, R.I., & Wiener, J.M. (2001, October) *Who will care for us?: Addressing the long-term care workforce crisis.* Washington, DC: The Urban Institute and American Association of Homes and Services for the Aging.

Straker, J.K. (2001, July). *Final report on survey development and testing for the Ohio nursing home resident satisfaction survey.* Oxford, OH: Miami University, Scripps Gerontology Center.

Sundstrom, E., De Meuse, K.P., & Futrell, D. (1990). Work teams: Applications and effectiveness. *American Psychologist, 45*(2), 120–133.

Susman, G.I. (1979). *Autonomy at work: A sociotechnical analysis of participative management.* New York: Praeger.

Talerico, K.A., & Evans, L.K. (2000). Making sense of aggressive/protective behaviors in persons with dementia. *The Gerontologist, 46,* 532.

Tannenbaum, S.I., Beard, R.L., & Salas, E. (1992). Team building and its influence on team effectiveness: An examination of conceptual and empirical developments. In K. Kelly (Ed.), *Issues, theory, and research in industrial organizational psychology.* New York: Elsevier.

Teresi, J.A., Holmes, D., Benenson, E., Monaco, C., Barrett, V., & Koren, M.J. (1993, December). Evaluation of primary care nursing in long-term care. *Research on Aging, 150*(4), 414–432.

Thomas, K.W., & Tymon, W.G. (1994). Does empowerment always work? *Journal of Management Systems, 6*(2), 1–13.

Thomas, K.W., & Velthouse, B.A. (1990). Cognitive elements of empowerment: An "interpretive" model of intrinsic task motivation. *Academy of Management Review, 15*(4), 666–681.

Thomas, W.H. (1994). *The Eden alternative: Nature, hope, and nursing homes.* Sherburne, NY: Eden Alternative Foundation.

Thomas, W.H. (2003). Evolution of Eden. In A.S. Weiner & J. Ronch (Eds.), *Culture change in long-term care* (pp. 141–158). New York: Haworth.

Thomas, W.H. (2006). *Eden alternative associate training.* Retrieved April, 1, 2006, from http://www.edenalt.com/associat.htm

Tjosvold, D. (1986). *Working together to get things done: Managing for organizational productivity.* Lexington, MA: Lexington.

Tuckman, B. (1965). Development sequence in small groups. *Psychological Bulletin, 63,* 384–399.

Uhlenberg, P. (1997). Replacing the nursing home. *The Public Interest, 182,* 73–80.

Varney, G. (1989). *Building productive teams: An action guide and resource book.* San Francisco: Jossey-Bass.

Veronesi, J. (2001). Home health integration for the future. *Home Health Care Management & Practice, 13*(4), 286–289.

Vickery, K. (1998). While stocks dry up, new financing options emerge for assisted living companies. *Provider.*

Vroom, V.H., & Yetton, P.W. (1973). *Leadership and decision-making.* Pittsburgh: University of Pittsburgh Press.

Wagner, D.L., Nadash, P., & Sabatino, C. (1997). *Autonomy of abandonment: Changing perspectives on delegation.* The National Council on the Aging. Retrieved May 3, 2000, from http://aspe.hhs.gov/daltcp/reports/autoabes.htm

Wagner, J.A. (1994). Participation's effects on performance and satisfaction. *Academy of Management Review, 19*(2), 312–330.

Wagner, L. (1998). Turning around turnover. *Provider, 24*(5), 71–72.

Waxman, H., Carner, E., & Berkenstock, G. (1984). Job turnover and job satisfaction among nursing home aides. *The Gerontologist, 24*(5), 503–509.

Weiner, A.S., & Ronch, J.L. (2003). *Culture change in long-term care.* New York: Harworth Social Work Practice Press.

Wellins, R.S., Byham, W.C., & Dixon, G. (1994). *Inside teams: How 20 world-class organizations are winning through teamwork.* San Francisco: Jossey-Bass.

Wellins, R.S., Byham, W.C., & Wilson, J.M. (1991). *Empowered teams: Creating self-directed work groups that improve quality, productivity, and participation.* San Francisco: Jossey-Bass.

Wetherbe, J.C. (1991, March). Executive information requirements: Getting it right. *MIS Quarterly,* pp. 51–65.

Whyte, H.L. (1995). Registered nurses' perceptions of empowerment and job satisfaction in a hospital setting. *JONA, 31,* 271.

Wiener, J. (2002). *Frontline long-term care worker project.* Washington, DC: The Urban Institute and the Institute for the Future of Aging Services.

Wiener, J., & Stevenson, D.G. (1998). *Long-term care for the elderly: Profiles of thirteen states* (Occasional Paper #12). Washington, DC: The Urban Institute.

Williams, K.J., & Alliger, G.M. (1994). Role stressors, mood spillover, and perceptions of work–family conflict in employed parents. *Academy of Management Journal, 37*(4), 837–868.

Wilner, M.A., & Wyatt, A. (1998). *Paraprofessionals on the front lines: Improving their jobs improving the quality of long-term care.* A conference background paper prepared for the AARP Long-Term Care Initiative by Paraprofessional Healthcare Institute, New York.

Wilson, K.B. (1994, January/February). Assisted living: A paradigm for consumers or a false hope. *Aging Today,* pp. 8–10.

Wilson, K.B. (1995). Assisted living as a model of care delivery. In L.M. Gamroth, J. Semradeck, & E.M. Tornquist (Eds.), *Enhancing autonomy in long-term care* (pp. 139–154). New York: Springer.

Wilson, K.B. (in press). Historical evolution of assisted living evolved in the United States, 1979–2003: Anchoring the research agenda with key concepts in the vision. *The Gerontologist.*

Wright, B. (2005). *Direct care workers in long-term care.* Washington, DC: AARP Public Policy Institute.

Wylde, M.A. (1998). *National survey of assisted living residents: Who is the customer?* Annapolis, MD: National Investment Conference for the Seniors Housing & Care Industries and Assisted Living Federation of America.

Yeatts, D.E., & Cready, C.M. (2007). Consequences of empowered CNA teams in nursing home settings: A longitudinal assessment. *The Gerontologist, 47,* 323–339.

Yeatts, D.E., Cready, C.M., Ray, B., DeWitt, A., & Queen, C. (2004). Self-managed work teams in nursing homes: Implementing and empowering nurse aide teams. *The Gerontologist, 44*(2), 256–261.

Yeatts, D.E., & Hyten, C. (1998). *High-performing self-managed work teams: A comparison of theory to practice.* Thousand Oaks, CA: Sage.

Yeatts, D.E., & Seward, R.R. (2000). Reducing turnover and improving health care in nursing homes. *The Gerontologist, 40*(3), 358–363.

Zey, M. (1992). *Decision making alternatives to rational choice models.* Newbury Park, CA: Sage.

Zimmerman, S., Gruber-Baldini, A.L., Sloane, P.D., Eckert, J.K., Hebel, J.R., Morgan, L.A., et al. (2003). Assisted living and nursing homes: Apples and oranges? *The Gerontologist, 43*(2), 107–117.

Zimmerman, S., Sloane, P.D., & Eckert., J.K. (2001). *Assisted living: Needs, practices, and policies in residential care for the elderly.* Baltimore: Johns Hopkins University Press.

Index